Fit & Fabulous

Elena Biedert

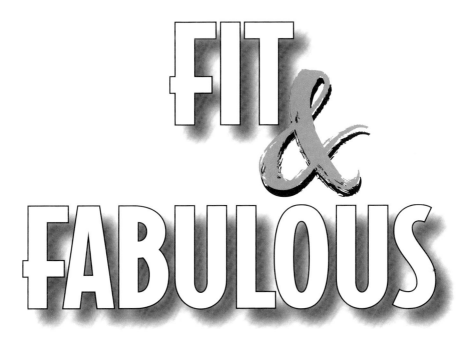

FIT & FABULOUS

12 Weeks to a Healthy, Confident, Happy You

 Intuitive Eating Plans

 Simple Workouts

 Achievable Goals

Meyer & Meyer Sport

British Library of Cataloguing in Publication Data

A catalogue record for this book is available from the British Library

Original title: *Einfach richtig fit werden*, © 2021 by Meyer & Meyer Verlag

Fit & Fabulous

Maidenhead: Meyer & Meyer Sport (UK) Ltd., 2024

ISBN: 978-1-78255-266-6

© 2024 by Meyer & Meyer Sport (UK) Ltd.

Aachen, Auckland, Beirut, Cairo, Cape Town, Dubai, Hägendorf, Hong Kong, Indianapolis, Maidenhead, Manila, New Delhi, Singapore, Sydney, Tehran, Vienna

 Member of the World Sport Publishers' Association (WSPA), www.w-s-p-a.org

Printed by Print Consult GmbH, Munich, Germany

Printed in Slovakia

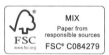

ISBN: 978-1-78255-266-6

Email: info@m-m-sports.com

www.thesportspublisher.com

CONTENTS

ACKNOWLEDGMENTS

The assumption that as a book author one is solely responsible for the creation of one's work seems plausible but has little to do with reality.

Even though in this book my own years of experience as a fitness enthusiast, trainer, and athlete have been carefully collected and presented, and I was the one who spent days and nights sitting on the manuscript, the success belongs to the whole team.

I would like to take this opportunity to thank everyone who contributed to the success of this book.

My thanks go to

- Robert Meyer, Alexa Deutz, and the rest of the team at Meyer & Meyer Sport for their active support.
- Tobias Serf for the beautiful and professional photos.
- Mareike Thelen for the flawless make-up and styling.
- Michael Wittig for the continuous inspiration and support.
- David Dückers for the impulse and kickstart.
- All my clients for their cooperation and experience, which went into the book.
- And finally, to my entire family, especially my husband and my son.

I could never have done it without all of you!

A heartfelt thank you also goes to you, dear reader. Thank you so much for your trust!

My additional thanks go to

- Liz Evans and the rest of the team at Meyer & Meyer Sport for believing in my work and making this English translation of my book a reality;
- Jana Short for mentoring me, her wisdom, and enabling my growth both as a professional and as an individual;
- Cassie Douglas for making me a better writer and for her valuable feedback on many of my articles and pitches;
- James Patrick for teaching me so much about the publishing culture during the past two years; and
- Kaged supplement brand and the whole team, who became like a family to me, for their continuous support, trust, and the "never stop evolving" energy.

To all of you, thank you!

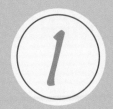

INTRODUCTION

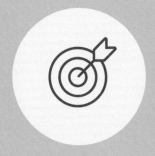

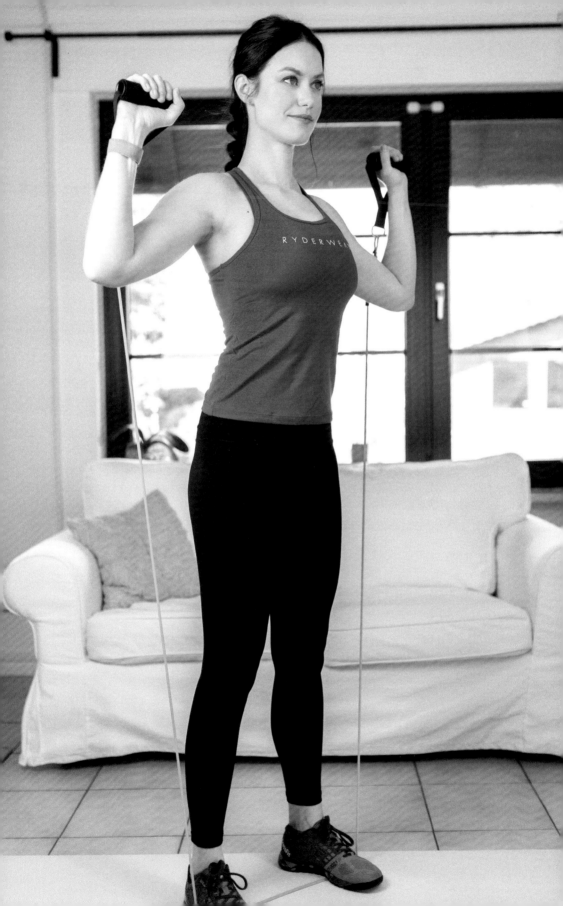

1 INTRODUCTION

Congratulations on your first step toward your dream figure and a healthier lifestyle. I am very happy that you have chosen this 12-week home workout program. And I hope you will have a lot of fun with it.

To guide you along the way, as you work your way through the program, you will receive several tips and recommendations from me. These will help you get the best results possible, no matter what your goal is.

Whether you want to lose weight, shape your body, or just work out for fun and health, this book will help you do it.

Since this 12-week program was created especially for those who can only work out from home, you won't need any big machines or expensive equipment to do it. However, you will need either an elastic fitness band (or a set of them) or a pair of dumbbells where you can screw the weight on or off. If you have both, all the better!

That said, this is not just a home workout program but a holistic guide that includes workouts, nutrition, as well as advice on everyday life and your attitude or mindset about working out. For all workouts or training sessions you need minimal equipment. This means that you can do them not only at home, but anywhere!

1.1 Equipment

Here are a few examples of the equipment for an optimal workout at home:

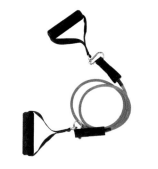

A set of elastic fitness bands with handles. You can combine different bands to make your workout more challenging.

Price range: *$15-$40, depending on the manufacturer.*

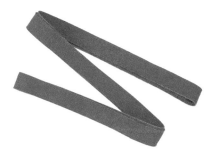

As an alternative to the bands with handles, you can get resistance bands. They are versatile and can be used to support pull-ups.

Price range: *$5-$40, depending on manufacturer and resistance level.*

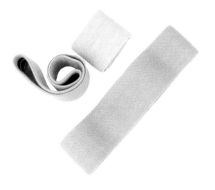

These short fabric bands, also known as booty bands, are perfect for training glutes. If you want to have round and tight glutes, these bands are essential for your arsenal.

Price range: *$10-$30, depending on the manufacturer for a whole set of three bands.*

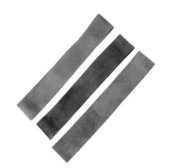

As an alternative to fabric bands, there are also elastic bands made of latex. However, these offer less resistance and can tear more quickly.

Price range: *$9-$20, depending on the manufacturer for a whole set.*

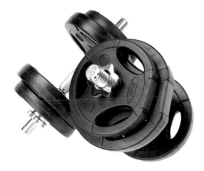

Optionally, you can get a set of adjustable dumbbells. These can help make your workout even more challenging. You can also combine the dumbbells with the bands.

Price range: *Starts at $45 for a 60 lb. adjustable dumbbell set.*

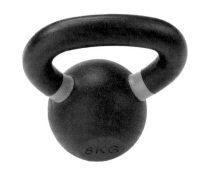

A kettlebell can also be used as an alternative. However, training with a kettlebell requires additional support, which is beyond the scope of this book.

Price range: *From $9, depending on weight and manufacturer.*

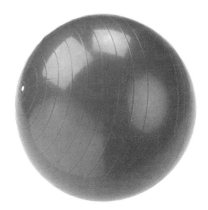

A Swiss ball is also perfect for training at home, and its use is often underestimated. You can use the ball for various exercises either as a training bench or to challenge your balance and core muscles.

Price range: *From $14, depending on manufacturer and size.*

My recommendation for this program is a set of elastic fitness bands with handles, an elastic band without handles with light or medium resistance, and a set of short fabric bands. If you also have some weights, that would be ideal.

However, if you don't have a fitness band or dumbbells at home, you can also use everyday household objects as additional weights for this program.

1.2 How should you work your way through the book?

In chapters 2 and 3, I will give you an overview of the entire training program. I will also explain how you can change your diet depending on your personal goal. Please read these two chapters carefully first. Make sure you understand everything and have everything you need for the next weeks.

Find a place where you can do your workouts in peace and set up your fitness bands or dumbbells and yoga mat there. Also do all the necessary shopping for your meals. If you want, you can prepare your meals for a day, a few days, or the whole week in advance.

The training program can be found in chapter 4. I recommend you do one week after the other, without skipping a certain week or changing the order. Please do all the training sessions and exercises in the order they are given. The whole program is designed to help you progress over time, get stronger, and achieve better results.

In chapter 5 we will recap what you have learned, and I will show you how to keep your progress going in the long run.

If there are any terms you don't know or if you want to better understand how to do a certain exercise step by step, you can read about it in section 7.2 and watch the corresponding instruction video.

I sincerely hope that you will enjoy the program! And always remember that you are capable of doing anything.

Have fun and best regards,

Elena Biedert
Certified fitness trainer, certified nutrition coach (ISSA International Sports Sciences Association), and coach for women and mothers.

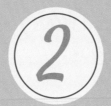

TRAINING PROGRAM OVERVIEW

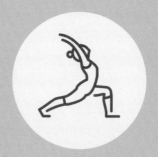

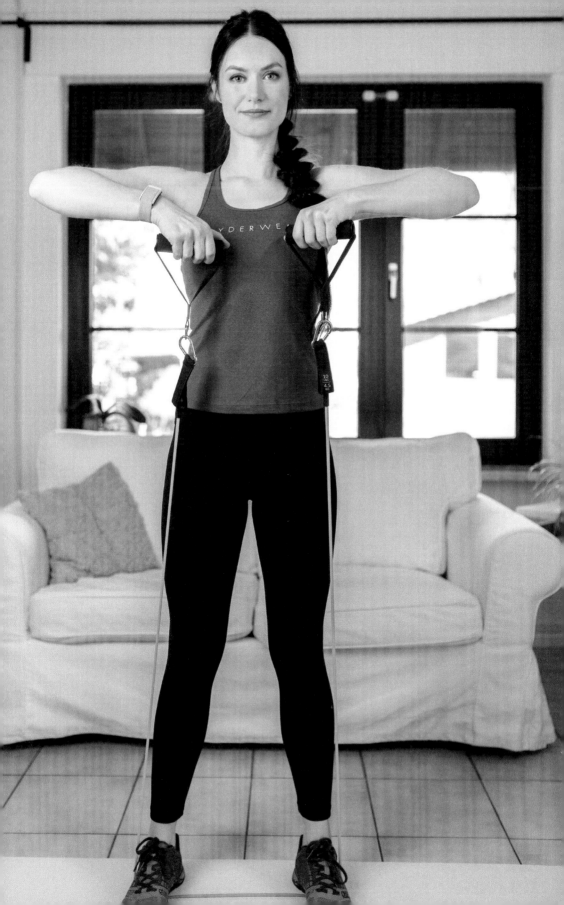

2 TRAINING PROGRAM OVERVIEW

The training program consists of three four-week phases. First, I will describe each phase individually in detail so you know exactly what to expect in the next 12 weeks.

2.1 Phase 1

This phase serves to create the required basics. If you have never trained before, you will be able to learn the relevant movements and exercises during this time. And if you already have some training experience, you can get used to the new program and, if necessary, improve your form and optimize your diet.

In Phase 1 you will do three training sessions per week, always training the whole body.

Your weekly schedule will look like this:

MONDAY	Full Body 1
TUESDAY	Rest Day
WEDNESDAY	Full Body 2
THURSDAY	Rest Day
FRIDAY	Full Body 3
SATURDAY	Rest Day
SUNDAY	Rest Day

2.2 Phase 2

During this phase we will continue to work on your strength. Your workouts will become more intense and challenging.

You will continue to train the whole body three times a week. In addition, you will have three days of active rest days. An active rest day means that you will not do any strength training that day, but you will try to stay active as much as possible.

For example, you could go for a jog, bike ride, walk, or swim for 20 minutes. Alternatively, if you don't feel like doing these or similar activities, I've prepared a quick workout for you for this day. This workout is not as intense as your other workouts, but it will still get you moving a bit.

Sunday, or the last day of your training week, is a rest day. This means you can just put your feet up and relax!

Your weekly schedule will look like this:

MONDAY	Full Body 1
TUESDAY	Active Rest Day
WEDNESDAY	Full Body 2
THURSDAY	Active Rest Day
FRIDAY	Full Body 3
SATURDAY	Active Rest Day
SUNDAY	Rest Day

NOTE

In all training phases, you don't necessarily have to start every Monday. You can choose the day that suits you best. However, do not change the order of the training sessions and always take a day off between your workouts in Phases 1 and 2.

2.3   Phase 3

Starting with this phase, we split the workouts between the lower body and the upper body. This gives us the opportunity to focus more precisely on specific muscle groups and eliminate possible weaknesses or imbalances, if there are any. You will do more workouts, and therefore your training routine will be more intense, but also more varied. Don't be afraid though, you can do it!

On the days you train your lower body, you will also do exercises for your abdomen.

The last four weeks will include between four and six workouts per week.

In fact, your workout will consist of four main workouts: two for your lower body and two for your upper body. If you prefer, you can focus solely on these workouts and still achieve good results.

However, in addition, you can add one or two more workouts if you want to focus on a specific muscle group or body part. In this program, we intentionally focus on the glutes and shoulders.

Why did I choose just these two body parts? As women, we often desire a narrow waist or a body that looks like an hourglass. However, the problem is that not everyone naturally has a slim waist. Some of us have a wider midsection, even if we have very little fat tissue. Some of us have wider shoulders and narrower hips. And some of us have narrow waists but equally narrow shoulders and hips. We are all so different!

With a specific workout and the right diet, we can – to a certain extent – shape our bodies the way we want them.

For example, if you have broader shoulders, then you could prioritize training your legs and glutes. In this way, you can change your lower body to look more proportionally balanced in relation to your upper body, making your waist look smaller.

If your midsection is genetically built to be a bit wider, you could make both your shoulders and your legs and glutes the focus of your workouts. This way, over time, you could get closer to the hourglass body shape, if that is your goal.

At this point, I want to make it clear that it's also perfectly fine if you're not aiming for a narrow waist or the typical "hourglass" physique! *The most important thing is that you feel comfortable in your own skin*. This can mean something completely different to everyone, and it doesn't necessarily have anything to do with looks or body type.

So, if you don't want to focus on your shoulders or glutes, simply disregard these specific workouts and engage in active rest on the selected days instead.

Your weekly schedule will look like this:

MONDAY	Lower Body 1 + Abs
TUESDAY	Upper Body 1
WEDNESDAY	Shoulders or alternatively Active Rest Day
THURSDAY	Lower Body 2 + Abs
FRIDAY	Upper Body 2
SATURDAY	Glutes or alternatively Active Rest Day
SUNDAY	Rest Day

NOTE

You don't necessarily have to start every Monday. You can choose the day that suits you best. However, do not change the order of the training.

TIP

If the training in the first phases is challenging and you also enjoy it, you can keep doing each phase for longer than four weeks before starting the next one. That said, to get good results, you should adapt the training to your capabilities. Read more about progression in chapter 4.

Join our private Facebook community: @MamaFitnessCoaching

Do you want to connect with like-minded people and quickly get support and answers to all the questions you might have about this book, this program, or nutrition and fitness in general? Then join our private Facebook community!

This group is aimed primarily at new moms and parents but welcomes all my clients, as well as anyone who would like to improve their fitness and diet. You will get access to helpful tips and resources, regular challenges, updates, exclusive previews, and so much more!

Looking forward to seeing you there!

Your coach, Elena

3

GUIDELINES FOR CHANGING YOUR DIET

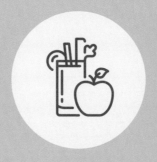

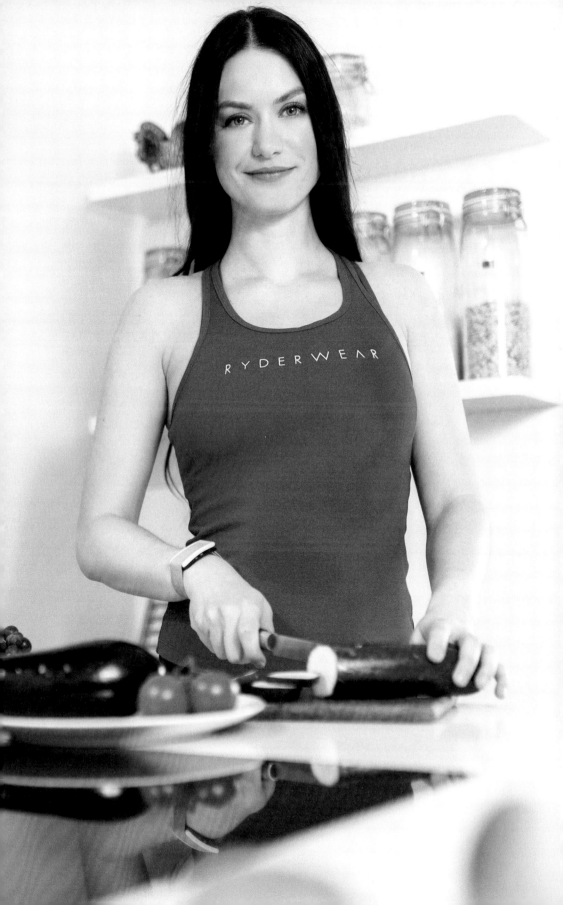

3 GUIDELINES FOR CHANGING YOUR DIET

If you don't want to train just for fun without a specific goal but rather to feel fit and comfortable in your skin, to change your body composition or shape in the long term, adequate nutrition matching your training is essential. If your diet is not in line with your goals, a workout program can often be a disappointment – you train so hard but see little or no progress.

For this program, I want to teach you the basics of a balanced diet in the simplest way possible. You won't find any extreme "diet tips and tricks" here, just general recommendations and a short guide on changing your diet in a healthy way for the long term without weighing your food or counting calories.

I will go into more detail about common possible goals – weight and fat loss, muscle gain, keeping the weight off, or just staying healthy. I will show you how to adapt your diet to each short- and long-term goal.

However, whatever your goal is, staying consistent and disciplined is essential. This may sound daunting at first – do you have to give up your whole social life now, all your favorite foods, and eat the same bland meals all the time?

The good news is that it doesn't have to be that way. To maintain your diet for as long as possible, it should be sustainable in the first place. Very strict "diets" often result in people giving up on them and a rebound because permanently giving up certain foods is unrealistic (Langeveld & de Vries, 2013; Ayyad & Andersen, 2000).

It also means that you should really enjoy your food. Always ask yourself if you feel good about what and how you eat.

- Can you imagine eating this way your whole life?

- Have you successfully achieved your goals this way without sabotaging yourself?

If your answer to these questions is "no," there are several ways to optimize your diet. However, it's up to you to decide what to do and how to do it. For example, if you like pasta and want to lose weight, you don't have to eat low-carb foods only and give up entirely on your favorite pasta. You know yourself best, and you alone can best decide which foods and meals you want or don't want to eat.

In this guide, you will not find a shopping list of "healthy products" that can lead to "black-and-white thinking". Some readers of this book might get the idea that the listed products are "good" and "healthy" while all others are "bad" or "unhealthy." This couldn't be further from the truth. Such "black-and-white thinking" tends to make our diet monotonous. However, our bodies need variety!

Instead of a strict shopping list, you'll get examples of different food groups, such as foods rich in protein, carbohydrates, fiber, or fats.

Again, these are just a few examples to give you some meal ideas. Regardless, you don't have to limit yourself only to these foods. You can eat anything you want. Really, anything! Instead of focusing on "good" and "bad", "healthy" and "unhealthy", pay attention to such things as **quality**, **portion size**, and your **eating habits**.

3.1 Basics of a healthy and balanced diet

3.1.1 Be mindful of what you eat and pay attention to your body

If you are mindful of what goes into your body, there is a very good chance that you will eat better. Think about what ends up in your shopping cart when you go grocery shopping or on your plate at every meal. Making mindful choices will automatically lead to better, well-thought-out decisions.

3.1.2 Focus on the quality of your food

Instead of relying mainly on industrially processed foods or pre-packaged meals, try to eat fresher, minimally processed, or completely unprocessed foods rich in macro- and micronutrients. However, this certainly doesn't mean that you should only buy organic produce from now on.

Instead of drinking orange juice, eat oranges. Instead of buying pre-made granola or cereals, buy oats and mix them with nuts, dried fruit, and cocoa.

Paying more attention to the quality of your food will significantly improve your diet and health.

Fresh, unprocessed products include a variety of grains, lentils, beans, fruits, vegetables, fresh meat, etc.

Minimally processed products include frozen berries, vegetables, fruits, canned tomatoes, canned tuna, etc.

Industrially processed products include pizza, burgers, frozen ready meals, ketchup, potato chips, etc. Almost all of these products have a very long list of ingredients on the package or are sold pre-cooked.

3.1.3 Vary your diet

Above all, eat a variety of foods to meet your nutritional needs. For example, you should have some protein with every meal. However, don't always eat just chicken breast. Instead, experiment with different types of meat, and include eggs, cheese, fish, lentils, tofu, and other protein-rich foods in your diet. There are many options to choose from, including vegetarian and vegan alternatives.

Add colorful fruits and vegetables to your daily menu. Also, focus on variety, or as it's often said, "Eat a rainbow!"

This means that you should always eat a mix of fruits and vegetables so your plate looks as colorful as a rainbow.

If your diet is not as diverse right now, try introducing one to two new foods to your weekly menu. Don't rush it, but implement small changes gradually. You can also consider taking an additional multivitamin, multimineral supplement, or omega-3 fatty acids.

3.1.4 Drink water

Water is essential for our metabolism and, thus, for all crucial processes in our body. Try to drink more water instead of sweetened beverages. Drink a glass of water when you get up in the morning and a glass of water with every meal.

Generally, you should drink 2-3 L (68-101 oz) or 30-40 mL of water per 1 kg of body weight, which is about 0.45-0.6 oz per 1 lb. of body weight. Yet, there is no specific information or recommendation regarding water consumption (Vivanti, 2012).

For example, if you weigh 54 kg (119 lb.), your water requirement could be 1.6-2.1 L or 53-71 oz per day. Note that our food contains water as well. If we eat a certain volume of fruit and vegetables daily, the water content consumed in our diet can be about 1 L.

If you are physically active, in a hot environment, drink alcohol, sweat a lot, have diarrhea, or feel very sick, your water or fluid requirement will increase accordingly.

3.1.5 Improve your eating habits

I've already mentioned the importance of mindful choices when grocery shopping. Becoming even more mindful of your eating habits will also improve your nutrition significantly.

1. Instead of rushing through your meal while watching your favorite show or scrolling on your phone, try focusing on the food itself. Eat slower, enjoying each piece that you put in your mouth. Notice the taste and texture of your dish.

2. Try to pay more attention to your body's cues. Are you actually that hungry? Or are you thirsty? Or maybe you are just bored? Or do you feel tired, stressed, or sad?

If you're simply bored, think about what you could do to keep yourself busy. If you're sad, call a friend, or watch something funny.

Ultimately, notice your true feelings and discover why you may feel hungry. After that, if you decide to eat something, you can still do it.

3. When you think you're getting full, stop eating.

4. Portion your meals according to your goals. We'll go into more detail about portioning below.

3.1.6 Learn how to cook and prepare your food

Learn how to prepare very simple and quick meals. Preferably ones you could take with you at any time, if necessary. Here are a few examples: classic chili or a variation of it, with boiled eggs, washed and chopped fruit and vegetables, salad with dressing, etc.

It is also a good idea to make a menu plan for the whole week, so you know exactly what you want to cook and when and can plan your shopping accordingly. Then only buy the foods you need for your menu.

Schedule when you want to cook and prepare your meals. Sometimes it saves a lot of time and stress if you have meals in your fridge that you have prepared in advance and are ready to eat. Unlike frozen pre-made meals, meals you cook yourself are rich and balanced in nutrients.

Cook for at least one day in advance. If your daily routine is very hectic, it might help to cook for a few days or even a whole week ahead. Then simply store the prepped meals in the refrigerator or freezer.

3.1.7 Avoid "black-and-white" thinking

There are no "good" and "bad" foods. Some foods are rich in macro- and micronutrients, while others are less nutritious. Make your choice: *Try to eat just a little bit better each day than the day before.*

For example, if you ate too much, don't blame yourself so that you become flooded with guilt. Instead, reduce the portion size of your next meal. If you "accidentally" ate an entire chocolate cake, try to understand why that happened.

*   Did you possibly eat too little protein that day?

*   Were you distracted while eating?

*   Or is something happening in your life right now that is keeping you emotionally charged?

Of course, eating that chocolate cake may have been a very conscious decision, and that's okay too. Try to be in tune with yourself and with your goals. Understand what drives you and try to make a slightly better choice next time.

3.1.8 Adapt your environment

If you keep convenience foods or sweets in your house, you are most likely to eat some or all of them. Likewise, if the people around you don't offer you support or don't understand your motivation, sooner or later, your plans will most likely be undermined, making reaching your goals impossible.

1. Try to clear out your kitchen by getting rid of the less nutritious foods. You should always have plenty of "healthier" alternatives in your house.

2. Find people who have the same interests as you. For example, join an online or a local community in your town, or sign up for a fitness class.

3. If your friends or family members don't support you, try to explain to them why a healthy and balanced diet is so important to you. Although it can sometimes be difficult, ask for their support. Also, make it clear that just because you're doing it, doesn't mean you're asking them to change their diet, too.

3.2 How to portion a meal

You can measure your meals in several ways: weigh your food and enter the data into an app, choose a smaller or a larger plate, or use your hands as a measuring tool. In this guide, I'll address the latter.

Unlike the commonly encouraged but often hated weighing of food and calorie counting, this portioning approach is intuitive, convenient, and easy to implement. We always have our hands with us, even when we eat in a restaurant or at a friend's house.

Also, our hands are usually proportional to our bodies: larger people need more food and tend to have larger hands. Smaller people need less food and smaller portions and typically have smaller hands.

Portioning with your hands is not only easy, but it also allows you to consume an optimal amount of nutrients per meal.

Assuming you usually eat four meals a day – breakfast, lunch, a snack in between, and dinner – include the following in each of your meals:*

- A serving of food high in protein that is the size of your palm (equivalent to about 20-30 g of protein).

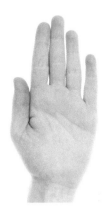

- A serving of food high in carbs the size of one cupped hand (equivalent to about 20-30 g of carbohydrates).

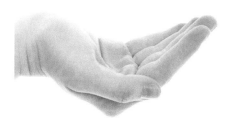

- A serving of vegetables the size of a fist.

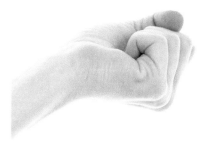

- A serving of food high in fats the size of one thumb (equivalent to about 7-12 g of fats).

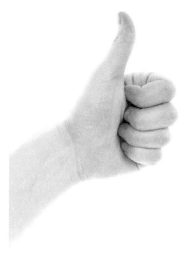

* For men, double these values.

3.2.1 Adapt these portions to your personal goal

Of course, everyone has their unique goal. For example, some would like to lose weight, while others would like to build muscle mass and change their body shape.

The above portioning guidelines are just a starting point. Try to eat this way for two weeks. See how your weight and appearance change, but keep in mind that our weight varies a lot from day to day. This depends on various factors and is absolutely normal!

Therefore, do not focus too much on the number on the scale.

Of course, the scale can be an important tool to reflect your transformation. And it works even better together with photos of you or your body measurements.

For example, you could take pictures of yourself every month, take body measurements every two weeks, and check your weight every week. You could also rely entirely on how you feel if that makes you more comfortable.

GOAL: LOSE WEIGHT

A classic diet goal is weight or fat loss. If this is your goal, portion all your meals as described above.

If you don't see any changes in your body after two weeks, reduce the portion of carbohydrates or fats. Remove half to one cupped hand of carbohydrates or half to one thumb of fat from one or two of your meals.

For men, double these values: reduce one to two cupped hands of carbohydrates or one to two whole thumbs of fat.

3.2.2 How much weight can I realistically lose and how fast?

How fast and how much body fat you can lose depends, among other things, on how consistently you follow the recommendations above. A realistic rate of weight loss per week is 0.4%-0.8% of your body weight.

For example, if your weight is 132 lb., expect to lose 0.5-1 lb. per week, and the less body fat you have, the slower the loss rate.

Note: Since our weight varies daily, as already mentioned, this refers to the average weekly weight. If we look at two weeks, for example, we get the following result (the considered weight is from Monday to Sunday and is in pounds):

Average weight change (lb.)

	Mo	Tu	We	Th	Fr	Sa	Su	Average (rounded)
Week 1	133.6	132.9	132.7	134	133.1	133.1	133.4	133.2
Week 2	133.4	132.9	133.6	132.3	133.4	132.9	132.7	133

This example shows a weight loss of about 0.2 lb. in one week. If you had only weighed yourself on Tuesdays, you would think you had made no progress. And if you had weighed yourself on Wednesdays only, you might be upset about the extra 0.9 lb.

Weighing yourself every day gives you more data to analyze. However, having more data is not always good or suitable for everyone. If you notice that you are focusing too much on the scale numbers and it is overwhelming for you, then weigh yourself only occasionally or use other methods to document your progress, such as photos, body measurements, or even your feelings that have nothing to do with your appearance (e.g., you're in a better mood, you can lift more weight, you finally have less pain in your back, etc.).

GOAL: GAIN MUSCLE MASS

Many women are often frightened by the idea of building muscles. They think this is not something a feminine woman does because they automatically think of bulky bodybuilders. However, this is a myth. On the contrary, a good muscle mass is the foundation for the often-desired toned and attractive female physique.

If you have been portioning all your meals as described above every day for two weeks but do not see any changes, then increase the portion of carbohydrates or fat.

Add half to one cupped hand of carbohydrates or half to one thumb of fat to one or two of your meals.

* For men, double these values: add one to two cupped hands of carbohydrates or one to two whole thumbs of fat.

3.2.3   How much muscle mass can I realistically build and how fast?

For women, this process is much slower than for men because of their hormone levels. A realistic rate of gain is 0.5% of body weight per month for beginners to only 0.19% of body weight per month for experienced female athletes. However, an actual figure varies from person to person and depends on several factors.

For example, if your weight is 132 lb., you could gain 0.6 lb. per month if you are just starting out, or only about 0.2 lb. per month if you are an advanced athlete.

Fat gain is inevitable if you want to gain muscle mass and shape your body. However, keep an eye on your body fat percentage and consider the above rate when gaining weight. When building muscle, sometimes we focus too much on the numbers on the scale and expect the number to keep going up. The danger with this is that you might not notice if you are gaining too much body fat if you get lost in the numbers.

3.3 What about supplements like protein powders and others? Are they absolutely necessary?

Supplements are exactly what their name implies: they simply supplement your diet. Whether you're just starting out with exercise or are already an experienced athlete, a balanced diet with a sufficient intake of macro- and micronutrients through food is always the priority.

If your diet is not that varied or you find it challenging to include certain foods or nutrients, like eating enough protein, you can consider taking some supplements.

Which supplements you need depends on various things. The best way to determine if you are deficient in specific vitamins or minerals is to get blood work done. For example, you could be vitamin D deficient if you rarely spend time in the sun.

If you rarely or never eat fish, it might make sense to supplement with omega-3 fatty acids.

And if you have a hard time getting protein into every meal, or maybe you have a stressful day and not enough time to cook, you could drink a protein shake.

That said, before relying on supplements, you should try to improve your diet with the help of the tips mentioned above.

3.4 Conclusion

In this chapter, I gave you all the tools you need. To help you avoid feeling lost and overwhelmed, I'll guide you through the entire program and show you how to change your diet step by step using my experience as a nutrition coach. I will start by addressing the areas commonly needing the most adjustments, which, if improved, would bring significant long-term benefits.

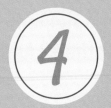

TRAINING PROGRAM

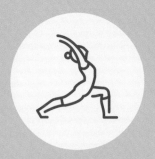

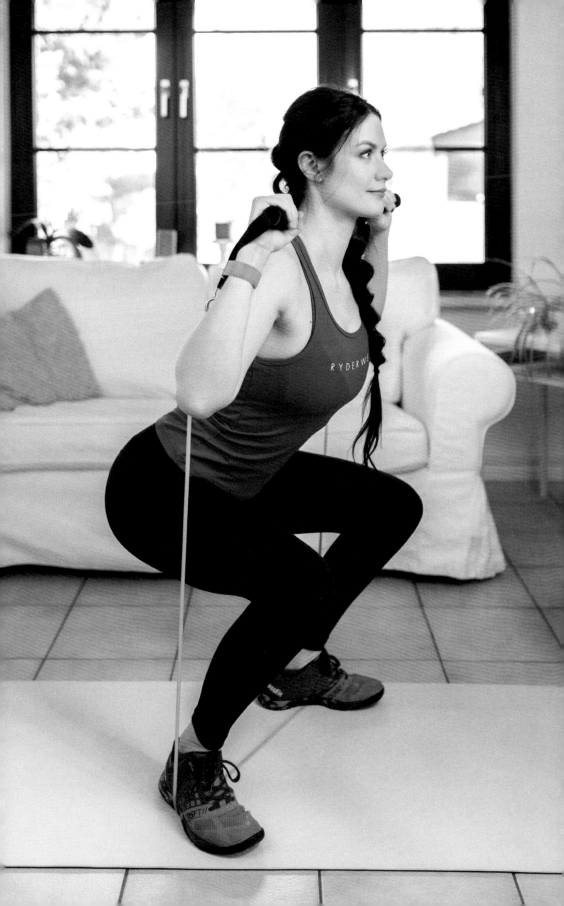

4 TRAINING PROGRAM

4.1 Phase 1

During the first four weeks, we will lay the foundations. If you have never trained before, you will learn the necessary movements and exercises during this time. And if you already have some training experience, you can use this time to familiarize yourself with the new program and, if necessary, improve your form and optimize your nutrition.

In Phase 1, you will do three training sessions per week, training the whole body in each session.

Your weekly schedule will look like this:

MONDAY	Full Body 1
TUESDAY	Rest Day
WEDNESDAY	Full Body 2
THURSDAY	Rest Day
FRIDAY	Full Body 3
SATURDAY	Rest Day
SUNDAY	Rest Day

NOTE

You don't necessarily have to start every Monday. You can choose the day that suits you best. However, do not change the order of the training sessions and always take a day off between your workouts.

Each training session is structured as follows:

1. You start with a warm-up, which prepares your body for the workout ahead. A warm-up is mainly about mobilizing the different joints and your spine and warming up the muscles. This helps you to work out more efficiently and reduces the risk of injury (Pérez-Gómez et al., 2020).

2. The warm-up is followed by the main workout block, which consists of various strength exercises. In Phase 1, we train the entire body in each training session.

3. The last block, after the main workout, is the cool-down. The goal is to come to rest after the strength training and to stretch and relax all muscles. Too often, this part is far too short, but it is not less important than the warm-up or the workout itself. The cool-down will help you speed up your recovery after a workout and reduce muscle soreness the next day. In addition, light stretching after physical activity can help you release tension and prevent the muscles from shortening. Thus, it can prevent various injuries (Apostolopoulos et al., 2018). If you don't have time, you can still quickly stretch the whole body or the muscles trained on that day. It doesn't have to be long because even a brief cool-down is much better than none at all!

4.1.1 WEEK 1

Welcome to your first training week! Before we start the program, I would like you to define your main goal as precisely as possible. You can do this as follows:

1. FIRST, UNDERSTAND WHAT EXACTLY YOU WANT

- What do you want? Lose weight or fat, build muscle mass, or just add some exercise to your daily routine and feel stronger?

- Do you want to see a certain number on the scale? What number do you want it to be? Do you realize how long it may take to reach that number (see section 3.2.1)?

- Do you want to achieve a particular physique? Which one exactly? What do you want to change? Is this realistic?

- Do you want to improve your diet? What exactly does that mean to you?

Keep asking yourself different questions until you have a clear vision of your goal and understand how long it might take to achieve it.

2. FIND YOUR TRUE MOTIVATION OR UNDERSTAND WHY YOU WANT TO DO THIS

You have defined and understood precisely what you want in the first step. Now it's time to uncover why you want it. To find out, you can use the "five whys" method. Believe me, the result can surprise you a lot.

The idea behind this method is to ask "Why?" at least five times, always basing your next question on the previous answer. Here is an example:

- "I would like to lose weight."

- *"Why do you want to lose weight?"*

- "I feel uncomfortable in my body and not attractive."

- *"Why do you feel unattractive?"*

- "My old clothes don't fit me, and I don't like what I see in the mirror when I'm not wearing clothes."

- *"Why is it so upsetting that you can't fit into your old clothes and don't like your reflection in the mirror with no clothes on?"*

- "My husband and I went out on dates much more often in the beginning of our relationship. Now we do much less together."

- *"Why does it bother you that you do less together?"*

- "It feels like there's not much spark between us anymore."

- *"And why does that bother you?"*

- "I miss our intimacy. I'm worried that my husband doesn't find me attractive anymore. And I want our relationship to go back to the way it was back then."

And now, within a few minutes, you have found your deeper and true motivation, your very own "Why." It is worth noting that you do not necessarily have to ask yourself "Why?" exactly five times. Keep asking until you find out the real reason behind your goal.

3. TRACK YOUR PROGRESS

If your goal is to change your body composition, lose weight, or shape your body, I recommend that you document where you are now before starting your training program. Even though it might be a struggle for you at first, believe me, you won't regret it later! It is always helpful to see where you started on the days when you don't feel as motivated. To do this, you can take the following measurements right after you get up and go to the bathroom but before you drink or eat anything:

- Use a scale to track your weight.

- Take body measurements with a measuring tape and note the circumference of your chest, waist, and hips. In addition, you can also measure the girth of your biceps, thighs, and calves on each side and your waist girth at the level of your belly button. This will give you a good understanding of your current state and any changes that will happen in the future.

- Take photos of yourself: Stand relaxed in front of the camera so you can be seen from head to toe, and take three pictures, one from the front, one from the side, and one with your back to the camera. Wear something light to make your body shape visible, such as a bikini or underwear. Here is an example of how you could take your photos:

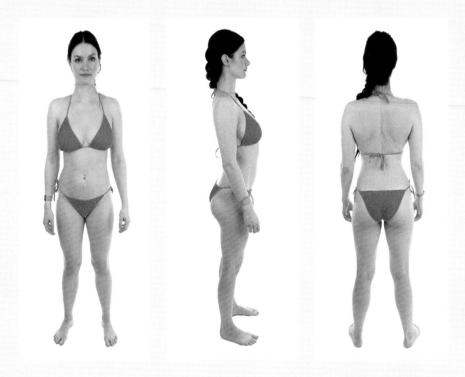

If you can or want to take only one of the measurements, that's fine too. However, you will have a more accurate picture of your progress if you have all three. I will tell you how to interpret them at the end of the program in section 5.1.

If your goal has nothing to do with your external appearance, I recommend keeping a kind of diary in which you can record your feelings, well-being, and actions or thoughts. For example, you can regularly write down what and how much you did on a particular day, how you felt that day or in a specific situation, what you ate that day, and so on. Because maybe you didn't reach the targeted number on your scale, but you feel more comfortable in your skin, stronger, and simply better. You shouldn't underestimate such little things!

MONDAY – FULL BODY 1

Congratulations on your first day of training! I hope you have set your goals and tracked your current stats (weight, body measurements, feelings, photos, etc.). Now let's get started with the workout!

NOTE

Throughout the book, I will use the notation "3 x 15." This means three sets of 15 repetitions per exercise. "5 reps each side" means one set of five repetitions for each side. "5 reps" represents one set of five repetitions.

WARM-UP (NO EQUIPMENT NEEDED)

 5 minutes

Your warm-up routine will not change during Phase 1 and Phase 2. Since you will be training the whole body, you should also prepare your entire body for the workout.

Please perform all movements slowly and in a controlled manner.

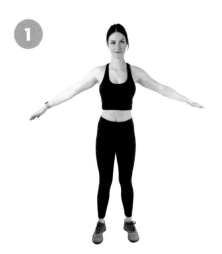

ARM CIRCLES *p. 304*
5 reps each direction
(forward and backward)

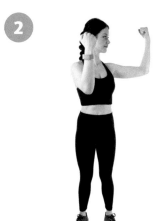

STANDING CHEST OPENER *p. 311*

5 reps each side

3

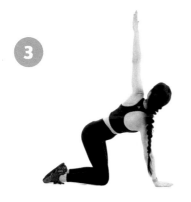

THREAD THE NEEDLE *p. 312*

3 reps each side

4

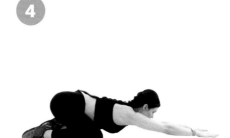

CHILD'S POSE ROCKING *p. 307*

10-15 seconds

5

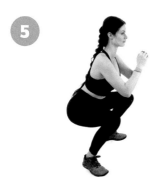

BODY WEIGHT DEEP SQUAT *p. 316*

5-10 reps

6

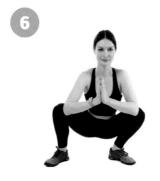

DEEP SQUAT WITH ANKLE
ROCKING *p. 309*

10-15 seconds while rocking from
one ankle to another

7

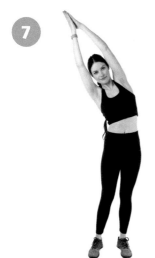

STANDING SIDE BEND *p. 315*

3 seconds each side

WORKOUT approx. 20 minutes

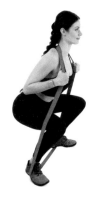

SQUAT *p. 271*
3 x 12

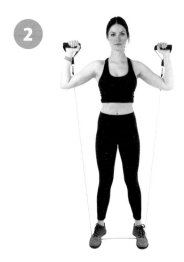

SHOULDER PRESS *p. 239*
3 x 12

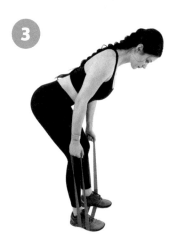

ROMANIAN DEADLIFT *p. 278*
2 x 12

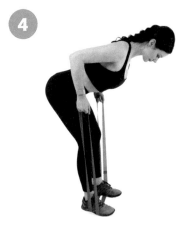

BENT-OVER ROW *p. 254*
3 x 12

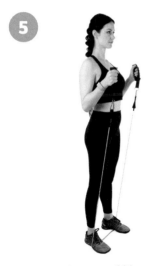

HAMMER CURL *p. 298*

2 x 15

NARROW PUSH-UP *p. 303*

2 x AMRAP

Rest between sets: 30 seconds.

AMRAP – as many reps as you can .

 5 minutes

COOL-DOWN

Your cool-down routine will not change during Phase 1 and Phase 2. After just a few workouts, you will master this routine in your sleep, allowing you to completely relax physically and mentally during the stretch.

The stretching program I'm about to share with you is my favorite routine, which I always do after my own workouts. I put it together myself many years ago and still enjoy it. It is a mix of different yoga poses, which flow from one pose to the next, along with simple stretches. I hope you will enjoy this routine as much as I do.

At first glance, the routine may seem complicated. However, once you understand the combination of the poses, it becomes very easy to remember the whole sequence.

You can decide for yourself how long you want to hold each position. If you want to have a quick stretch after your workout, you can just hold each position for one to five seconds. Let the transitions be slow and controlled.

If you have more time and want to stretch thoroughly, you can hold the positions as long as you like. In this case, let the poses flow into each other in a slow and controlled manner.

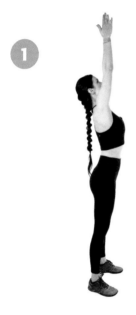

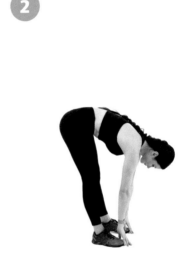

MOUNTAIN TO UPWARD SALUTE POSE *p. 325*
While inhaling

Stand straight and try to reach the ceiling with your hands.

STANDING FORWARD BEND (UTTANASANA) *p. 328*
While exhaling

Bend forward to stretch the back of your thighs.

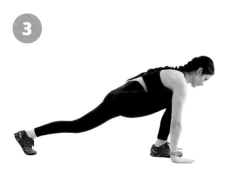

3

HIGH LUNGE (ONE SIDE) *p. 320*
While inhaling

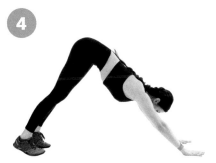

4

DOWNWARD FACING DOG *p. 317*
While exhaling

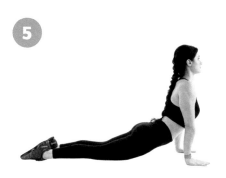

5

UPWARD FACING DOG *p. 318*
While inhaling

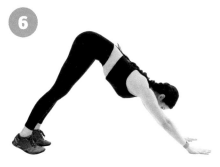

6

DOWNWARD FACING DOG *p. 317*
While exhaling

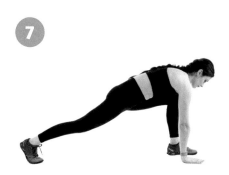

7

HIGH LUNGE (OPPOSITE SIDE) *p. 320*
While inhaling

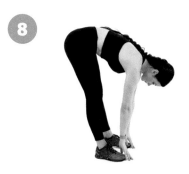

8

STANDING FORWARD BEND
(UTTANASANA) *p. 328*
While exhaling

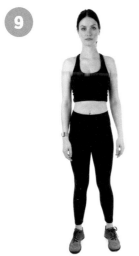

MOUNTAIN TO UPWARD
SALUTE POSE *p. 325*
While inhaling

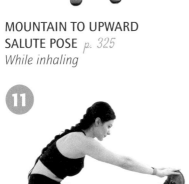

SEATED FORWARD BEND *p. 321*

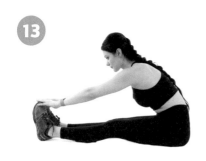

REPEAT 11 *p. 321*

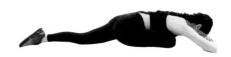

PIGEON TO HALF PIGEON POSE
TO SINGLE-LEG FORWARD BEND
POSE *p. 326*
One side

REPEAT 10 FOR THE
OPPOSITE SIDE *p. 326*

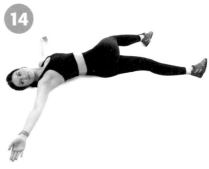

SUPINE SPINAL TWIST
Each side *p. 323*

Here you can find the video of the cool-down sequence that includes exercises 1-9.

Here you can find the video of the cool-down sequence that includes exercises 10-13.

TUESDAY – REST DAY

Today is your rest day, so please take a rest!

YOUR NUTRITION

This week is all about observing. Write down everything you eat and drink, including all snacks, sauces, and oils for cooking and frying. Really, absolutely everything that you put into your mouth. It would be awesome if you could do this all week. However, you could alternatively just take three representative days, such as two weekdays and one weekend day.

This is how you can keep a record of your meals:

Meal Diary

Time	What and how much did you eat or drink?	Note
8:30	A cup of black coffee, unsweetened, two slices of whole grain bread, one slice of salami, and one slice of light cheese.	I didn't have much time and was very tired

WEDNESDAY – FULL BODY 2

 ## WARM-UP (NO EQUIPMENT NEEDED)   5 minutes

Repeat the warm-up from Monday: Full Body 1, *pp. 44–45.*

 ## WORKOUT   approx. 20 minutes

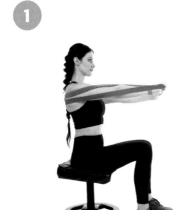

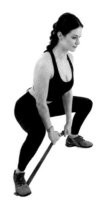

SEATED CHEST PRESS *p. 245*
2 x 12

SUMO SQUAT *p. 282*
3 x 12

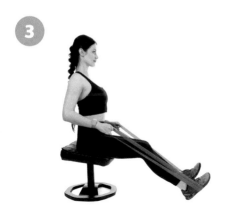

SEATED ROW *p. 252*
3 x 15

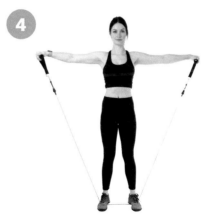

LATERAL RAISE *p. 240*
3 x 12

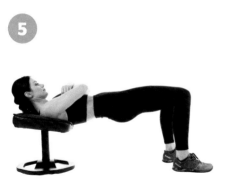

HIP THRUST *p. 290*
3 x 12

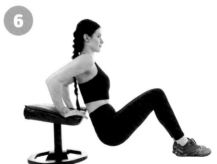

COUCH OR CHAIR DIP *p. 300*
2 x 10

Rest between sets: 30 seconds.

 5 minutes　　　　　　　　COOL-DOWN　

Repeat the cool-down from Monday: Full Body 1, *p. 48.*

THURSDAY – REST DAY

Today is your rest day, so please take a rest!

INTERESTING FACT

Did you know that digestion begins in the brain, not the stomach? When we see or think about food, our brain tells the rest of the body to prepare for eating (Gropper, Smith & Groff, 2009).

FRIDAY – FULL BODY 3

 WARM-UP (NO EQUIPMENT NEEDED)   **5 minutes**

Repeat the warm-up from Monday: Full Body 1, *pp. 44–45.*

 WORKOUT   **approx. 20 minutes**

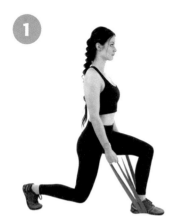

REVERSE LUNGE *p. 265*
3 x 12 each side

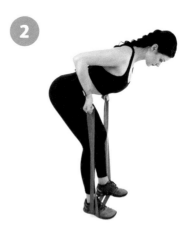

BENT-OVER ROW WITH SUPINATED GRIP *p. 255*
3 x 12

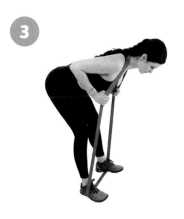

GOOD MORNING *p. 295*
2 x 12

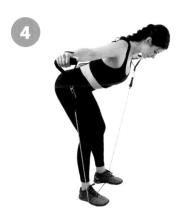

BENT-OVER LATERAL RAISE *p. 241*
3 x 12

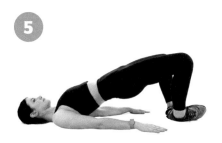

FROG PUMP *p. 294*
2 x 30

ELBOW PLANK *p. 263*
2 sets, hold each set as long as you can

Rest between sets: 30 seconds.

 5 minutes   COOL-DOWN

Repeat the cool-down from Monday: Full Body 1, *pp. 48-50.*

SATURDAY AND SUNDAY – REST DAYS

Your first training week is over, and you can finally take some time to recover. Recovery and rest are important to your progress, so take them as seriously as your training. Today and tomorrow are your rest days: recover and relax!

Your second training week starts on Monday, but now you can look back at the first week and review it:

* How was it for you?

* How was your nutrition so far? Compare what you ate with the information from chapter 3. Is there anything you can do better next week? If so, what exactly?

* For the next week, pick just one thing you can do better and try to do it consistently. I suggest you start with appropriate protein portioning.

4.1.2 WEEK 2

The workouts this week are the same as in week 1, but now, when you are more familiar with the exercises, we will adjust the number of repetitions in each exercise. If you are training with dumbbells, you can use the same weight as last week.

If the last repetition of each set feels too easy, try adding more resistance or weight. The last repetition in each set must be challenging but still doable with a good execution form.

It is important that you achieve some sort of progression from week to week. Also known as "Progressive Overload," it means the continuous increase of the intensity of your workouts, and this refers to the increase of the stress placed upon your body.

Progressive Overload is essential to make progress and is achievable through many different ways: by increasing the number of repetitions; increasing the weight; changing the amplitude of movement with the same weight; or training with the same weight but faster and more explosively. Also, with Progressive Overload, progress can be happening despite losing body fat/weight. The program is already built in such a way that you progress from week to week.

YOUR NUTRITION

As mentioned above, try to eat an optimal amount of protein this week. A good starting point is to include a palm-sized portion of protein-rich foods in each meal. For example, if you eat four times a day, see section 3.2. If you eat only three times a day, you can divide this amount accordingly, for example, one and a half palm-sized portions for breakfast, one portion for lunch, and one and a half palm-sized portions for dinner.

You can start with only two adjusted meals to make it easier for you. In other words, you portion only two meals according to the instructions and eat the rest as usual. Try to have all your meals with adjusted protein portions by Sunday at the latest.

To help you keep track of your portions, you will find a table to fill out at the end of each week.

MONDAY – FULL BODY 1

 ## WARM-UP (NO EQUIPMENT NEEDED)   5 minutes

Repeat the warm-up from last Monday: Full Body 1, *pp. 44–45.*

 ## WORKOUT   approx. 20 minutes

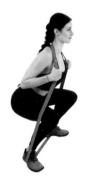

SQUAT *p. 271*
3 x 15-20

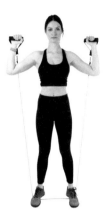

SHOULDER PRESS *p. 239*
3 x 15-20

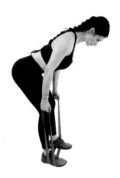

ROMANIAN DEADLIFT *p. 278*
2 x 15-20

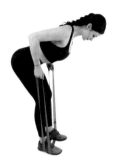

BENT-OVER ROW *p. 254*
3 x 15-20

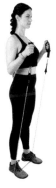

HAMMER CURL *p. 298*
2 x 15

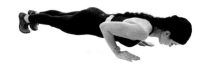

NARROW PUSH-UP *p. 303*
2 x AMRAP

Rest between sets: 30 seconds.

 5 minutes

COOL-DOWN

Repeat the cool-down from last Monday: Full Body 1, *pp. 48–50.*

TUESDAY – REST DAY

Today is your rest day, so please take a rest!

INTERESTING FACT

Many people eat oranges when they want to get an extra boost of vitamin C. Did you know, though, that broccoli and red bell peppers contain much more vitamin C than an orange?

As an example:

100 g of broccoli contains 89 mg of vitamin C, and 100 g of red bell pepper has 127 mg of vitamin C.

In contrast, 100 g of oranges contain only 53 mg of vitamin C.
(US Department of Agriculture, 2019)

WEDNESDAY – FULL BODY 2

 WARM-UP (NO EQUIPMENT NEEDED)   **5 minutes**

Repeat the warm-up from last Monday: Full Body 1, *pp. 44–45.*

 WORKOUT   **approx. 20 minutes**

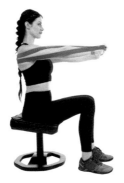

SEATED CHEST PRESS *p. 245*
2 x 15-20

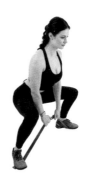

SUMO SQUAT *p. 282*
3 x 15-20

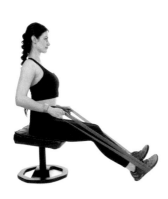

SEATED ROW *p. 252*
3 x 15-20

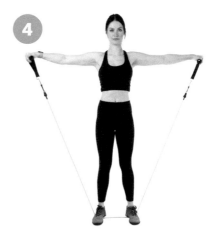

LATERAL RAISE *p. 240*
3 x 15-20

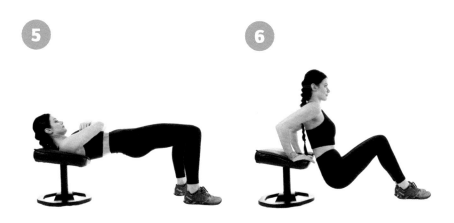

HIP THRUST *p. 290*
3 x 20

COUCH OR CHAIR DIP *p. 300*
2 x 15

Rest between sets: 30 seconds.

 5 minutes

COOL-DOWN

Repeat the cool-down from last Monday: Full Body 1, *pp. 48–50.*

THURSDAY – REST DAY

Today is your rest day, so please take a rest!

INTERESTING FACT

A cup of coffee could be just as effective as an expensive fat-burning supplement. Regardless of what you take, no fat will be burned if you do not perform physical activity (Astrup et al., 1990).

FRIDAY – FULL BODY 3

 ## WARM-UP (NO EQUIPMENT NEEDED)   **5 minutes**

Repeat the warm-up from last Monday: Full Body 1, *pp. 44–45.*

 ## WORKOUT   **approx. 20 minutes**

This Friday, you will do the Side Plank instead of the Elbow Plank like last week.

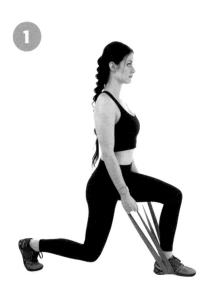

1

REVERSE LUNGE *p. 265*
3 x 15 each side

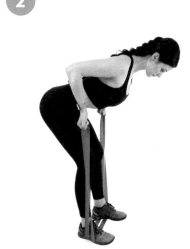

2

BENT-OVER ROW WITH SUPINATED GRIP *p. 255*
3 x 15-20

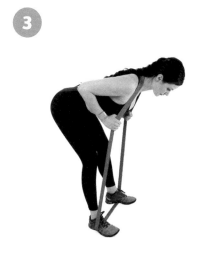

GOOD MORNING *p. 295*
2 x 15-20

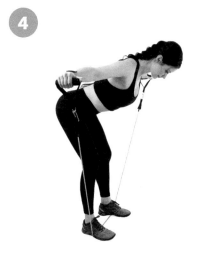

BENT-OVER LATERAL RAISE *p. 241*
3 x 15

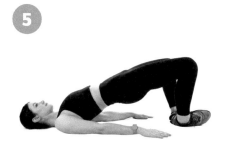

FROG PUMP *p. 294*
2 x 30

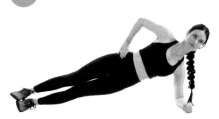

SIDE PLANK *p. 262*
2 sets each side, hold each set
as long as you can.

Rest between sets: 30 seconds.

 5 minutes COOL-DOWN

Repeat the cool-down from last Monday: Full Body 1, *pp. 48–50.*

SATURDAY AND SUNDAY – REST DAYS

• Now you can recover and review the past week.

• How were your training and nutrition so far?

• What is the greatest achievement you've had?

In the following table, you can mark how many portions of protein you ate each day. Just cross out the circles.

Track daily protein intake

	Protein	Carbs	Fats	Veggies	Water*
Required portions per day	4				
Monday	○○○○				
Tuesday	⊘⊘⊘○				
Wednesday	○○○○				
Thursday	⊘⊘⊘○				
Friday	○○○○				
Saturday	⊘⊘⊘○				
Sunday	○○○○				

*Please enter your own quantity, considering the recommendations.

Next week we will adjust the portions of carbohydrates and fats in your meals.

4.1.3 WEEK 3

This week some new exercises have been added.

Do all exercises slower: three to four seconds eccentric phase and one to two seconds concentric phase. For example, the eccentric phase is when you give in to the resistance when you squat. The concentric phase is when you resist by contracting your muscles, for example, when you stand up from a squat.

If possible, slightly increase the weight or resistance this week.

YOUR NUTRITION

This week, we're trying to adjust the amount of carbohydrates and fats in your meals. Assuming you eat four meals a day, try to include a cupped hand of foods rich in carbohydrates and a thumb of foods rich in fats in each of your meals (see section 3.2).

You can distribute this amount accordingly if you eat less often or more than four times a day.

To make it easier for you, start with only two adjusted meals. In other words, you portion out only two meals according to the above instructions and eat the remaining meals as usual. Try to have adjusted the portions of carbohydrates and fats in all your meals by Sunday at the latest. The protein portions should be already adapted for all meals from the beginning of the week.

If one day doesn't go perfectly for you, that's totally fine. Just try to do better the next day. What counts is how consistent you are over a longer period. Don't fall into the "black-and-white" or "all-or-nothing" mindset.

To help you keep track of your portions, you'll find a table at the end of the week.

MONDAY – FULL BODY 1

 ## WARM-UP (NO EQUIPMENT NEEDED)   **5 minutes**

Repeat the warm-up from Week 1, Monday: Full Body 1, *pp. 44–45.*

 ## WORKOUT   **approx. 20 minutes**

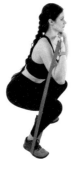

FRONT SQUAT *p. 274*
3 x 15-20

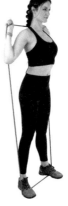

BEHIND-THE-NECK PRESS *p. 238*
3 x 15-20*

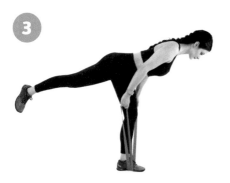

SINGLE-LEG DEADLIFT *p. 267*
2 x 12-15 each side

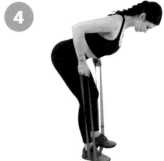

BENT-OVER ROW *p. 254*
3 x 15-20

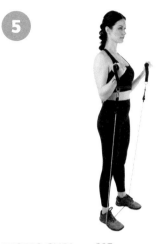

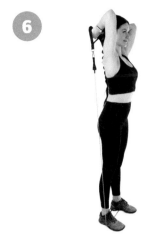

BICEPS CURL *p. 297*
2 x 15

OVERHEAD TRICEPS
EXTENSION *p. 301*
2 x 12-15

Rest between sets: 30 seconds.

* If your flexibility is limited and you find this exercise difficult, you can do regular shoulder press instead of behind-the-neck press.

 5 minutes   COOL-DOWN

Repeat the cool-down from Monday: Full Body 1, *pp. 48–50.*

TUESDAY – REST DAY

Today is your rest day, so please take a rest!

INTERESTING FACT

Even though the exercise itself is a stressor, low- or moderate-intensity workouts can sometimes help you relieve stress and speed up your recovery. A casual walk, meditation, or yoga are good examples (Kellmann, 2010).

WEDNESDAY – FULL BODY 2

 WARM-UP (NO EQUIPMENT NEEDED)   5 minutes

Repeat the warm-up from Monday: Full Body 1, *pp. 44–45.*

 WORKOUT   approx. 20 minutes

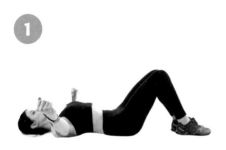

FLY *p. 246*
2 x 12-15

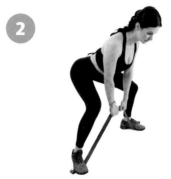

SUMO DEADLIFT *p. 283*
3 x 15-20

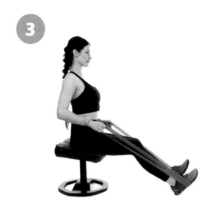

SEATED ROW *p. 252*
3 x 15-20

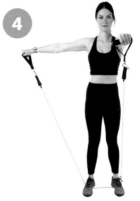

**ALTERNATING FRONT AND
LATERAL RAISE** *p. 234*
3 x 16-20

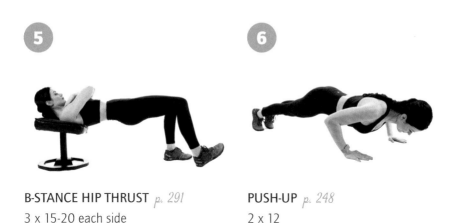

B-STANCE HIP THRUST *p. 291*
3 x 15-20 each side

PUSH-UP *p. 248*
2 x 12

Rest between sets: 30 seconds.

 5 minutes

COOL-DOWN

Repeat the cool-down from Monday: Full Body 1, *pp. 48–50.*

THURSDAY – REST DAY

Today is your rest day, so please take a rest!

Enjoy your day, read a book, or take a short walk outside.

FRIDAY – FULL BODY 3

 WARM-UP (NO EQUIPMENT NEEDED)   5 minutes

Repeat the warm-up from Monday: Full Body 1, *pp. 44–45.*

 WORKOUT   approx. 20 minutes

1

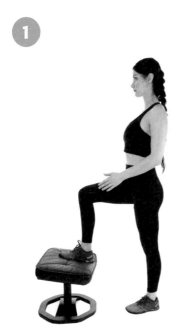

STEP-UP *p. 281*
3 x 15 each side

2

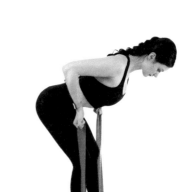

BENT-OVER ROW WITH
SUPINATED GRIP *p. 255*
3 x 15

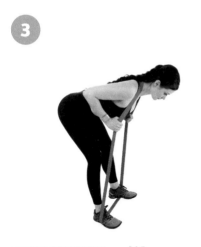

GOOD MORNING *p. 295*
2 x 15

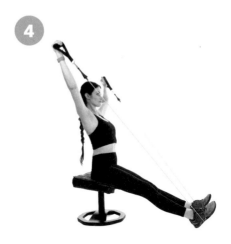

SEATED Y RAISE *p. 244*
3 x 10-12

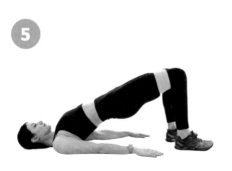

BANDED GLUTE BRIDGE *p. 285*
2 x 30

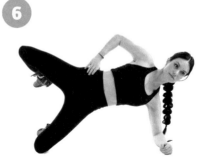

SIDE-LYING HIP RAISE *p. 279*
2 x 10-15 each side

Rest between sets: 30 seconds.

 5 minutes   **COOL-DOWN**

Repeat the cool-down from Monday: Full Body 1, *pp. 48–50.*

SATURDAY AND SUNDAY – REST DAYS

- Now you can recover and review the past week.

- How were your training and nutrition so far?

- What is the greatest achievement you've had?

In the following table, you can mark how many portions of protein, carbs, and fats you ate each day. Just cross out the circles.

Track the daily intake of protein, carbs, and fats.

	Protein	Carbs	Fats	Veggies	Water*
Required portions per day	4	4	4		
Monday	○○○○	○○○○	○○○○		
Tuesday	○○○○	○○○○	○○○○		
Wednesday	○○○○	○○○○	○○○○		
Thursday	○○○○	○○○○	○○○○		
Friday	○○○○	○○○○	○○○○		
Saturday	○○○○	○○○○	○○○○		
Sunday	○○○○	○○○○	○○○○		

Please enter your own quantity, considering the recommendations.

Next week we will adjust the vegetable in your meals.

4.1.4 WEEK 4

This week's workouts are the same as in Week 3, but we will adjust the number of repetitions in the exercises. Notice how the number of repetitions varies depending on what type of equipment or resistance you use: a resistance band, dumbbells, or another kind of weight where you can change the load or resistance.

This week, try to choose resistance so that the last repetition of each set feels very challenging. However, the execution form should always remain correct.

YOUR NUTRITION

This week, we'll try incorporating lots of vegetables into your diet. Assuming you eat four meals a day, try to eat a fist-sized portion of vegetables at each meal (see section 3.2).

You can distribute them accordingly if you eat less frequently or more frequently than four times a day.

Remember not to change everything immediately and start with only two adjusted meals first. That means you portion only two meals according to the instructions above and eat the remaining meals as usual. Try to have modified vegetable portions in all your meals by Sunday at the latest. Your protein, carb, and fat amounts should ideally be portioned appropriately for all meals at the beginning of the week.

Also, pay attention to how much water you drink. The recommended *minimum* fluid intake is 30-40 mL per kg of body weight or about 0.45-0.6 oz per 1 lb. However, this amount will increase if, for example, you regularly engage in intensive exercise. A good indicator is the color of your urine – if the color is slightly yellow or almost clear, then you are drinking enough. You should drink a lot, although not so much that you have to go to the bathroom every 15-30 minutes.

To help you keep track of your portions, you will find a table at the end of the week.

MONDAY – FULL BODY 1

 ## WARM-UP (NO EQUIPMENT NEEDED) 5 minutes

Repeat the warm-up from Monday: Full Body 1, *pp. 44–45.*

 ## WORKOUT approx. 20-25 minutes

 ### RB = RESISTANCE BAND, DB = DUMBBELL

If none of the labels are present, it means that you are performing this repetition number regardless of the equipment you are using. Adjust the resistance or weight appropriately.

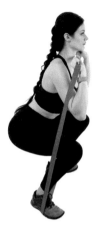

FRONT SQUAT *p. 274*
3 x 18-20 (RB) / 15 (DB)

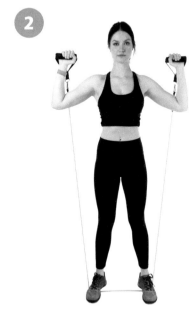

SHOULDER PRESS *p. 239*
3 x 18-20 (RB) / 15 (DB)

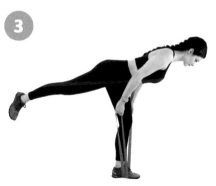

SINGLE-LEG DEADLIFT *p. 267*
2 x 18-20 (RB) / 12 (DB), each side

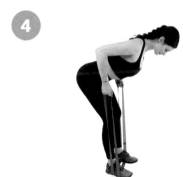

BENT-OVER ROW *p. 254*
3 x 15-20

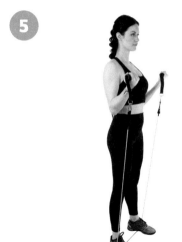

BICEPS CURL *p. 297*
2 x 15

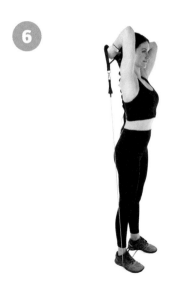

OVERHEAD TRICEPS EXTENSION *p. 301*
2 x 15

Rest between sets: 30-45 seconds.

 5 minutes　　　　　　　　COOL-DOWN

Repeat the cool-down from Monday: Full Body 1, *p. 48–50.*

TUESDAY – REST DAY

Today is your rest day, so please take a rest!

INTERESTING FACT

A common myth is that you should not eat any carbs in the evening before going to bed, or you will gain weight.

However, it is the weekly average of calorie intake that determines whether you lose or gain weight or fat. When exactly you eat is secondary. This means you can even eat a whole cake before sleeping without gaining weight. Just make sure you consume the right number of calories throughout the week and the appropriate distribution of nutrients throughout the day (Hill et al., 2018).

WEDNESDAY – FULL BODY 2

WARM-UP (NO EQUIPMENT NEEDED)

 5 minutes

Repeat the warm-up from Monday: Full Body 1, *pp. 44–45.*

WORKOUT

 approx. 20-25 minutes

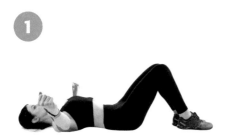

FLY *p. 246*
2 x 15

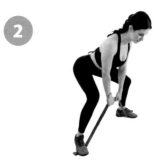

SUMO DEADLIFT *p. 283*
3 x 18-20 (RB) / 15 (DB)

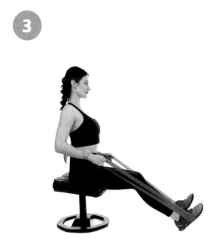

SEATED ROW *p. 252*
3 x 15

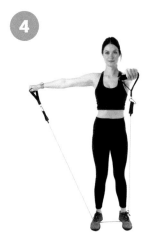

ALTERNATING FRONT
AND LATERAL RAISE *p. 234*
3 x 16 (RB) / 12-14 (DB)

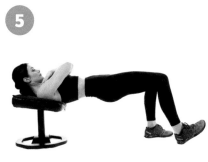

B-STANCE HIP THRUST *p. 291*
3 x 20 (RB) / 12 (DB), each side

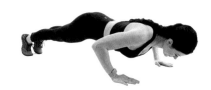

PUSH-UP *p. 248*
3 x 10

Rest between sets: 30-45 seconds.

 5 minutes

COOL-DOWN

Repeat the cool-down from Monday: Full Body 1, *p. 48–50.*

THURSDAY – REST DAY

Today is your rest day, so please take a rest!

FRIDAY – FULL BODY 3

 WARM-UP (NO EQUIPMENT NEEDED)   **5 minutes**

Repeat the warm-up from Monday: Full Body 1, *pp. 44–45.*

 WORKOUT   **approx. 20-25 minutes**

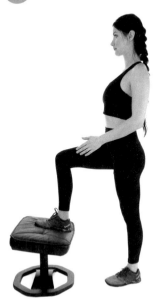

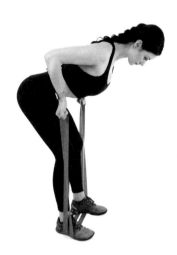

STEP-UP *p. 281*
3 x 15 each side

**BENT-OVER ROW WITH
SUPINATED GRIP** *p. 255*
3 x 15-20

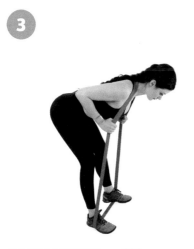

GOOD MORNING *p. 295*
2 x 15-20

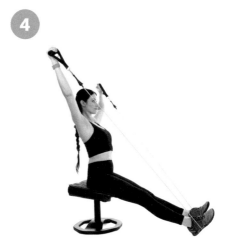

SEATED Y RAISE *p. 244*
3 x 12

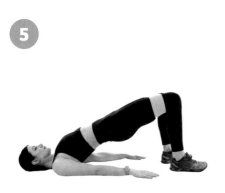

BANDED GLUTE BRIDGE *p. 285*
2 x 30

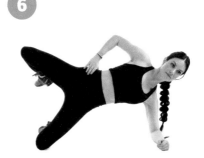

SIDE-LYING HIP RAISE *p. 279*
2 x 10-15 each side

Rest between sets: 30-45 seconds.

 5 minutes

COOL-DOWN

Repeat the cool-down from Monday: Full Body 1, *pp. 48–50.*

INTERESTING FACT

Here are six possible reasons why your weight fluctuates from day to day:

- You ate more salt than usual. Your body holds more water as a result.

- You have eaten more carbohydrates than usual. Carbohydrates in the form of glycogen are stored together with water in the body, namely 3 g of water for every 1 g of glycogen.

- You have to go to the bathroom.

- You had a heavy training session the day before. Because of the microtrauma in your muscles, you might store more water.

- Your period is supposed to start soon. Hormones affect many processes in our body, and weight fluctuations around your period are perfectly normal.

- You are just a human being! So many internal processes in our bodies and external factors, such as sleep and stress, can affect the weight on your scale.

Weight fluctuations are normal and do not automatically mean fat or muscle. More often than not, it is just water. Keep an eye on the weight trend over weeks or calculate the weekly average weight to be sure (Baker & Norton, 2019).

SATURDAY AND SUNDAY – REST DAYS

Now you can recover and review the past week.

- How were your training and nutrition so far?

- What is the greatest achievement you've had?

In the following table, you can mark how many portions of protein, carbs, fats, and vegetables you ate each day. Just cross out the circles.

Track the daily intake of protein, carbs, fats, vegetables, and the amount of water intake.

	Protein	Carbs	Fats	Veggies	Water*
Required portions per day	4	4	4	4	
Monday	○○○○	○○○○	○○○○	○○○○	
Tuesday	●●●●	●●●●	●●●●	●●●●	
Wednesday	○○○○	○○○○	○○○○	○○○○	
Thursday	●●●●	●●●●	●●●●	●●●●	
Friday	○○○○	○○○○	○○○○	○○○○	
Saturday	●●●●	●●●●	●●●●	●●●●	
Sunday	○○○○	○○○○	○○○○	○○○○	

*Please enter your own quantity

You will check your progress on Monday morning and adjust your diet accordingly.

4.2 Phase 2

During this phase we will continue to work on your strength. Your workouts will become more intense and challenging.

You will continue to train the whole body three times a week. In addition, you will have three active rest days. An active rest day means that you will not do any strength training that day, but you will try to stay active as much as possible.

For example, you could go for a jog, bike ride, walk, or swim for 20 minutes. Alternatively, if you don't feel like doing these or similar activities, I've prepared a quick workout for you for this day. This workout is not as intense as your other workouts, but it will still get you moving a bit.

Sunday, or the last day of your training week, is a rest day. This means you can just put your feet up and relax!

Your weekly schedule will look like this:

MONDAY	Full Body 1
TUESDAY	Active Rest Day
WEDNESDAY	Full Body 2
THURSDAY	Active Rest Day
FRIDAY	Full Body 3
SATURDAY	Active Rest Day
SUNDAY	Rest Day

Your training sessions are structured as in Phase 1: You always start with a warm-up to prepare your body for the upcoming workout. After the warm-up, you start the main workout, followed by the cool-down.

The warm-up and cool-down remain the same as in Phase 1.

NOTE

You don't necessarily have to start every Monday. You can choose the day that suits you best. However, do not change the order of the training sessions and always take a day off between your workouts.

4.2.1 WEEK 5

For the next four weeks, you will train your whole body in a single session, just as you did in the last phase. However, your training sessions will be more intense because you will train with *supersets* in this second phase.

A superset consists of two exercises performed one after the other without rest. Suppose a superset consists of exercises A and B, each with three sets and 15 repetitions. In that case, this means that you first perform a set of 15 repetitions of exercise A and then a set of 15 repetitions of exercise B without resting in between.

That would be one set in your superset. After finishing one superset, you can take the rest as stated in your workout. After the rest, you start the second set of the superset and so on until you have finished all supersets.

Starting this week, you will also start doing some new exercises. Remember that you can always look up the exact execution form and instructions in section 7.2.

This week, try to choose such resistance so that the last repetition of each set feels very challenging. However, the execution form should always remain technically correct.

PROGRESS MONITORING

Before starting the training week, we need to check your progress first. As described before the first week, you can weigh yourself, take your body measurements, and take your progress photos. Always do this in the morning right after you get up and after you have been to the bathroom but before eating or drinking anything.

Even if it's hard sometimes, try not to let the numbers and pictures affect you too much. Treat this check-in simply as a data input. Be curious about what else you can make out of it!

After you have gathered all your data, you need to interpret it. Think again about your goal and what you want to achieve. Is it slowly going in the right direction (see section 3.2.2)?

If things start going in the right direction, don't change anything for now. Just continue to follow the same diet as before. Of course, if you can improve something, such as eating less processed products or being more mindful of your diet, you can focus on that. But don't change your portion sizes.

That said, if things aren't going according to your plan, find out how you can optimize your diet (see chapter 3).

MONDAY – FULL BODY 1

 WARM-UP (NO EQUIPMENT NEEDED) **5 minutes**

Repeat the warm-up from Monday: Full Body 1, *pp. 44–45.*

 WORKOUT **approx. 20 minutes**

SUPERSET 1:

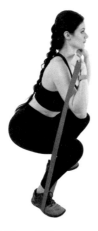

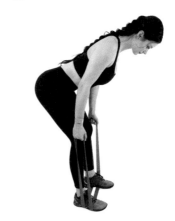

FRONT SQUAT *p. 274*
3 x 15

ROMANIAN DEADLIFT *p. 278*
3 x 15

SUPERSET 2:

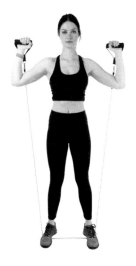

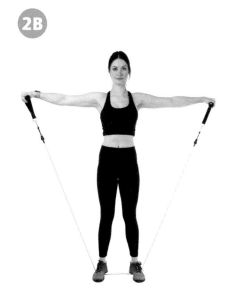

SHOULDER PRESS *p. 239*
3 x 15

LATERAL RAISE *p. 240*
3 x 15

SUPERSET 3:

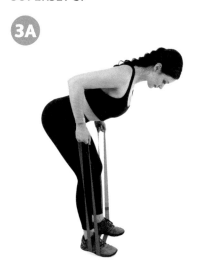

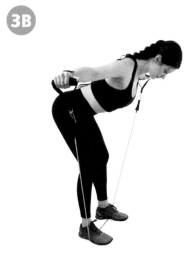

BENT-OVER ROW *p. 254*
3 x 15

BENT-OVER LATERAL RAISE *p. 241*
3 x 15

SUPERSET 4:

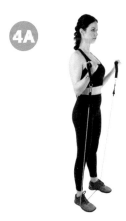

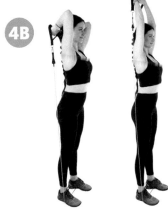

BIZEPS-CURL *p. 297*

2 x 15

OVERHEAD TRICEPS
EXTENSION *p. 301*

2 x 15

Rest between supersets: 30-45 seconds.

COOL-DOWN

 5 minutes

Repeat the cool-down from Monday: Full Body 1, *pp. 48-50.*

TUESDAY – ACTIVE REST DAY

The goal on this day is to stay active as much as possible, along with a light cardio exercise.

Here are some examples of activities you could do:

- Ride your bike
- Go inline or roller skating
- Go for a walk
- Swim
- Jog.

Choose something you enjoy and exercise at 60%-70% of your maximum heart rate for 15-20 minutes.

The rule of thumb for determining your maximum heart rate is the following equation: HR_{max} (maximum heart rate) = 220 – age.

Example:

If you are 30 years old, your maximum heart rate is about 190 beats per minute.

60 % of HR_{max} 190 = 0.6 * 190 = 114

70 % of HR_{max} 190 = 0.7 * 190 = 133

This means that during the 15-20 minutes of training, your heart rate should stay between 114 and 133 beats per minute.

If you don't have a heart rate monitor or strap available, you can tell the proper intensity by the fact that you sweat slightly during the activity but can still talk.

As an additional option, you can do a quick circuit workout. You don't need any equipment or a gym for this.

Below you will find a sample circuit. You should do all six exercises one after the other in the given order without a break. After a short rest, you can repeat the circuit once or twice.

Try to do the movements as fast as possible, but always make sure that the exercise is performed correctly.

CIRCUIT 1

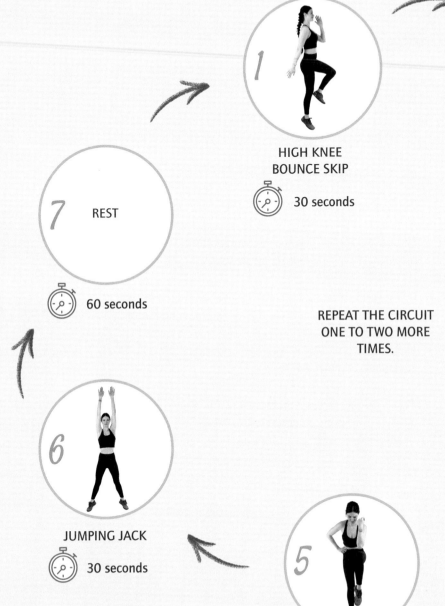

**HIGH KNEE
BOUNCE SKIP**

30 seconds

REPEAT THE CIRCUIT
ONE TO TWO MORE
TIMES.

7 REST

60 seconds

6

JUMPING JACK

30 seconds

5

**STANDING ELBOW-TO-KNEE
CRUNCH** (opposite side)

30 seconds

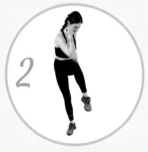

**STANDING OPPOSITE
ELBOW-TO-KNEE CRUNCH**
(one side)

 30 seconds

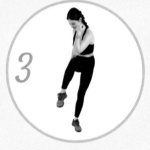

**STANDING OPPOSITE
ELBOW-TO-KNEE CRUNCH**
(opposite side)

 30 seconds

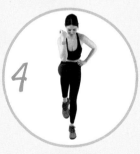

**STANDING
ELBOW-TO-KNEE CRUNCH**
(one side)

 30 seconds

WEDNESDAY – FULL BODY 2

 WARM-UP (NO EQUIPMENT NEEDED)   5 minutes

Repeat the warm-up from Monday: Full Body 1, *pp 44–45.*

 WORKOUT   **approx. 25-30 minutes**

Sumo means that your feet are placed wider than shoulder width.

SUPERSET 1:

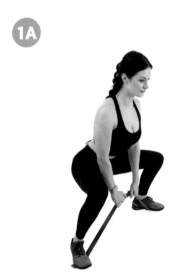

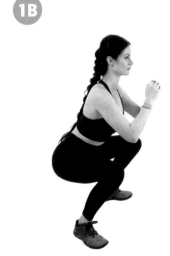

SUMO SQUAT *p. 282*
3 x 15

JUMP SQUAT *p. 268*
3 x 10

SUPERSET 2:

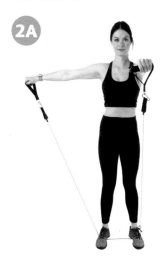

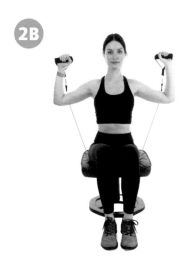

ALTERNATING FRONT AND
LATERAL RAISE *p. 234*
3 x 14

SEATED SHOULDER
PRESS *p. 239*
3 x 15

SUPERSET 3:

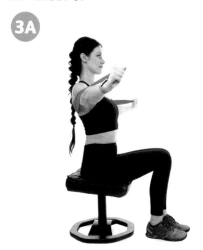

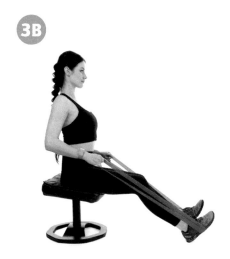

SEATED FLY *p. 247*
3 x 15

SEATED ROW *p. 252*
3 x 15*

SUPERSET 4:

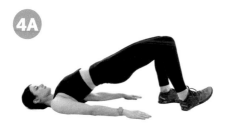

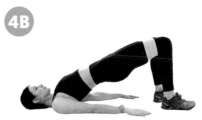

B-STANCE GLUTE BRIDGE *p. 284*
3 x 20 each side

BANDED GLUTE BRIDGE *p. 285*
3 x 20 **

* Hold the contraction for about 0.5-1 seconds until you release the band and straighten your arms.

** Hold the contraction for about 0.5-1 seconds until you lower your hips.

Rest between supersets: 30-45 seconds.

COOL-DOWN

 5 minutes

Repeat the cool-down from Monday: Full Body 1, *pp. 48-50.*

THURSDAY – ACTIVE REST DAY

See "Tuesday - Active Rest Day" of this week, *pp. 88-91.*

FRIDAY – FULL BODY 3

 5 minutes   WARM-UP (NO EQUIPMENT NEEDED)

Repeat the warm-up from Monday: Full Body 1, *pp. 44–45.*

 approx. 20-25 minutes   WORKOUT

SUPERSET 1:

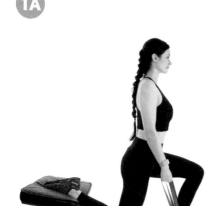

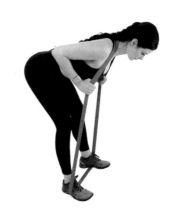

BULGARIAN SPLIT SQUAT *p. 266*
3 x 15 each side

GOOD MORNING *p. 295*
3 x 15

SUPERSET 2:

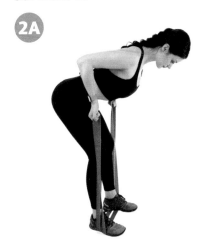

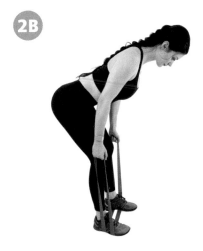

BENT-OVER ROW WITH SUPINATED GRIP *p. 255*

3 x 15

ROMANIAN DEADLIFT *p. 278*

3 x 15

SUPERSET 3:

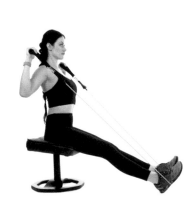

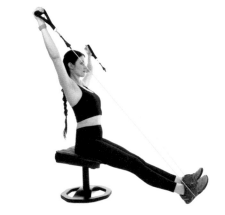

SEATED W ROW *S. 242*

3 x 15*

SEATED Y RAISE *p. 244*

3 x 5*

SUPERSET 4:

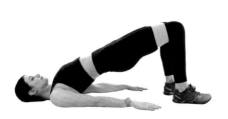

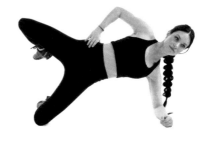

BANDED GLUTE BRIDGE *p. 285*
3 x 20**

SIDE-LYING HIP RAISE *p. 279*
3 x 10-15 each side **

*   *Hold the contraction for about 0.5-1 seconds until you release the band and straighten your arms.*

**   *Hold the contraction for about 0.5-1 seconds until you lower your hips.*

Rest between supersets: 30-45 seconds.

 5 minutes
COOL-DOWN

Repeat the cool-down from Monday: Full Body 1, *pp. 48–50.*

SATURDAY – ACTIVE REST DAY

See "Tuesday – Active Rest Day" of this week, *pp. 88–91.*

SUNDAY – REST DAY

Now you can finally rest and review the past week:

- How were your training and nutrition so far?
- What is the greatest achievement you've had?

In the following table, you can continue to keep track of your food and fluid intake. Since you should have adjusted the amount of protein, carbohydrates, and fats from the beginning of this week, please enter your own values.

Track the daily intake of protein, carbs, fats, vegetables, and the amount of water intake.

	Protein*	Carbs*	Fats*	Veggies*	Water*
Required portions per day					
Monday					
Tuesday					
Wednesday					
Thursday					
Friday					
Saturday					
Sunday					

*Please enter your own quantity

Next week, continue to eat the same portion sizes as this week.

Don't worry if this hasn't worked perfectly for you yet. Always remember that the goal is not to be perfect 100% of the time but to achieve long-term results. Every little thing counts because all those "little things" result in a significant change. Therefore, focus on being better tomorrow than you are today, both in your training and diet. And try to follow this approach every day.

4.2.2 WEEK 6

This week's workouts are similar to Week 5, but we will add some new exercises. You can find the exercise descriptions in section 7.2.

Try to choose such resistance so that the last repetition of each set feels very challenging. However, the execution form should always remain technically correct.

NUTRITION

Your nutrition remains the same as last week, but you can make small improvements every day. For example, choose one or two products you eat regularly but start consuming them in a less processed or unprocessed variation instead (e.g., eat an orange every day instead of drinking orange juice).

MONDAY – FULL BODY 1

 ## WARM-UP (NO EQUIPMENT NEEDED)   5 minutes

Repeat the warm-up from Monday: Full Body 1, *pp. 44–45.*

 ## WORKOUT   approx. 25-30 minutes

SUPERSET 1:

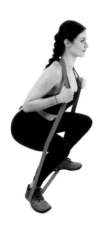   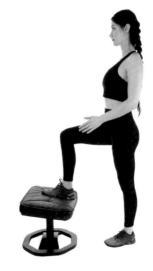

SQUAT *p. 271*   STEP-UP *p. 281*
3 x 15   3 x 15 each side

SUPERSET 2:

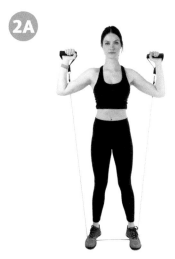

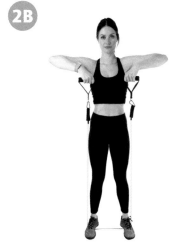

SHOULDER PRESS *p. 239*
3 x 15

UPRIGHT ROW *p. 236*
3 x 15

SUPERSET 3:

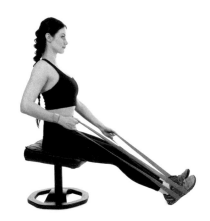

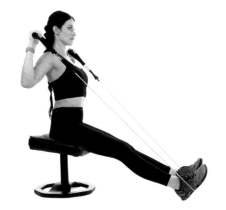

SINGLE-ARM ROW *p. 250*
3 x 15 each side

SEATED W ROW *p. 242*
3 x 15

SUPERSET 4:

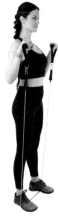

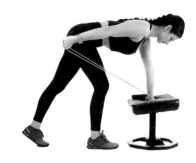

BICEPS CURL WITH PRONATED GRIP *p. 299*
2 x 15

TRICEPS KICKBACK *p. 302*
2 x 10-15 each side

Rest between supersets: 30-45 seconds.

COOL-DOWN

  5 minutes

Repeat the cool-down from Monday: Full Body 1, *pp. 48–50.*

TUESDAY – ACTIVE REST DAY

See "Tuesday - Active Rest Day" from Week 5, *pp. 88–91.*

Following, I'll give you another example of circuit training focusing on the abdominal muscles. You should perform all six exercises in a row in the given time without a break. After a short rest, you can repeat the circuit for one or two more rounds.

Try to do the movements as fast as possible, but always make sure that the exercise is performed correctly.

CIRCUIT 2

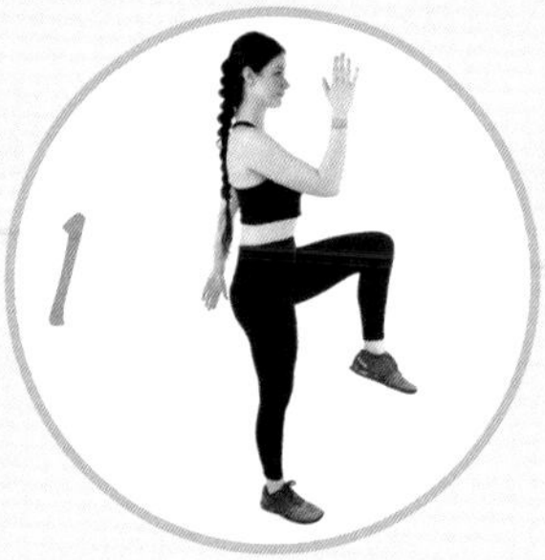

High Knees

30 seconds

7 REST

60 seconds

REPEAT THE CIRCUIT ONE TO TWO MORE TIMES.

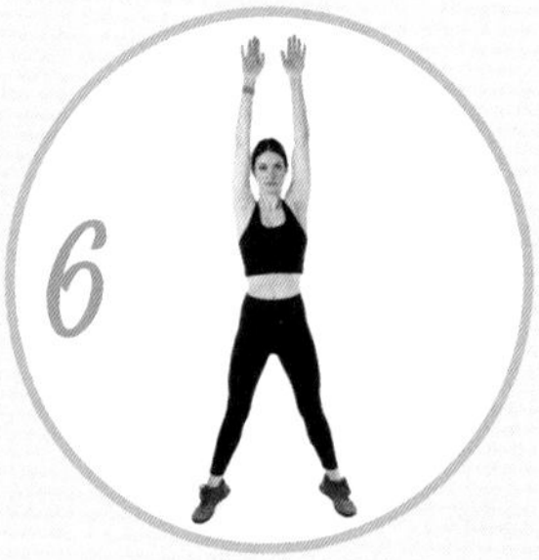

6

JUMPING JACK

30 seconds

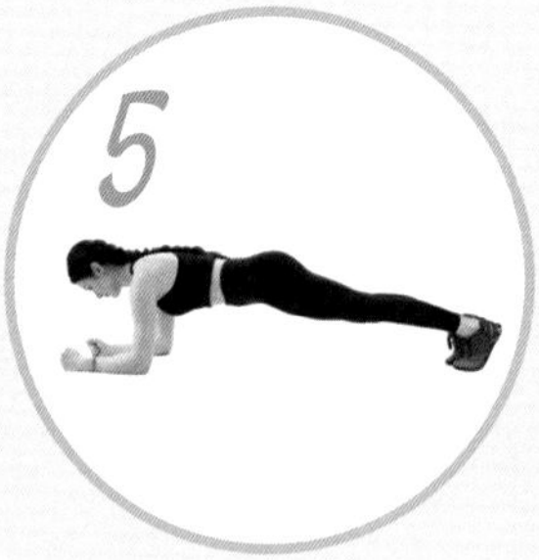

5

ELBOW PLANK

30 seconds

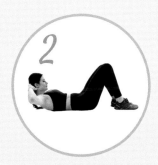

CRUNCH

 30 seconds

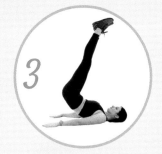

REVERSE CRUNCH

 30 seconds

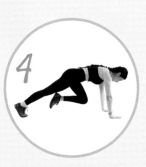

MOUNTAIN CLIMBER

 30 seconds

WEDNESDAY – FULL BODY 2

 ## WARM-UP (NO EQUIPMENT NEEDED)   **5 minutes**

Repeat the warm-up from Monday: Full Body 1, *pp. 44–45.*

 ## WORKOUT   **approx. 30-35 minutes**

SUPERSET 1:

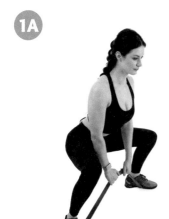

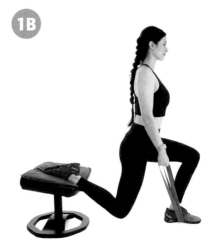

SUMO SQUAT *p. 282*
3 x 15

BULGARIAN SPLIT SQUAT *p. 266*
3 x 15 each side

SUPERSET 2:

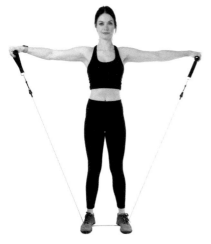

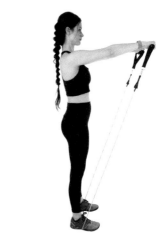

LATERAL RAISE *p. 240*
3 x 15

FRONT RAISE *p. 237*
3 x 15

SUPERSET 3:

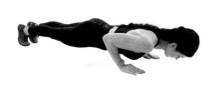

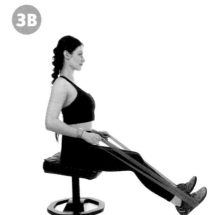

NARROW PUSH-UP *p. 303*
3 x 15

SEATED ROW *p. 252*
3 x 15*

SUPERSET 4:

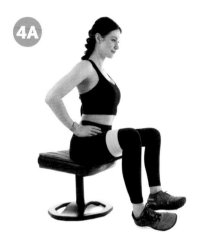

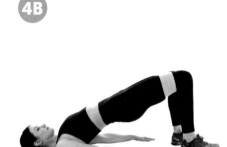

THREE-WAY SEATED BANDED HIP ABDUCTION (STRAIGHT UP/LEANING BACK/LEANING FORWARD) *p. 288*
3 x 20 / 20 / 20

BANDED GLUTE BRIDGE *p. 285*
3 x 20 **

*   *Hold the contraction for about 0.5-1 seconds until you release the band and straighten your arms.*

**   *Hold the contraction for about 0.5-1 seconds until you lower your hips.*

Rest between supersets: 30-45 seconds.

 ## COOL-DOWN

 5 minutes

Repeat the cool-down from Monday: Full Body 1, *pp. 48–50.*

THURSDAY – ACTIVE REST DAY

See "Tuesday – Active Rest Day" of this week, *pp. 103–105* or "Tuesday – Active Rest Day" from Week 5, *pp. 88–91.*

FRIDAY – FULL BODY 3

 5 minutes   **WARM-UP (NO EQUIPMENT NEEDED)**

Repeat the warm-up from Monday: Full Body 1, *pp. 44–45.*

 approx. 20-25 minutes   **WORKOUT**

SUPERSET 1:

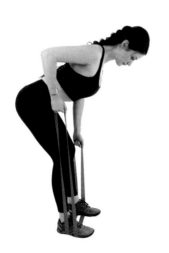

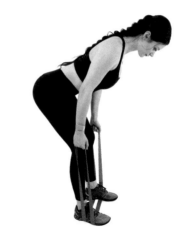

BENT-OVER SINGLE-ARM ROW *p. 253*
3 x 20 each side

ROMANIAN DEADLIFT *p. 278*
3 x 15-20

SUPERSET 2:

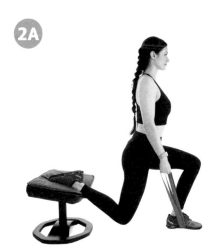

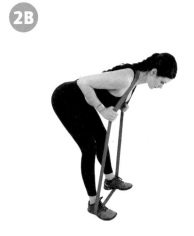

BULGARIAN SPLIT SQUAT *p. 266*
3 x 15 each side

GOOD MORNING *p. 295*
3 x 15

SUPERSET 3:

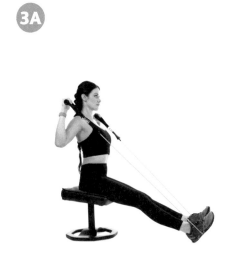

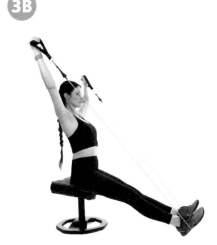

SEATED W ROW *p. 242*
3 x 15 *

SEATED Y RAISE *p. 244*
3 x 5 *

SUPERSET 4:

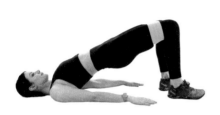

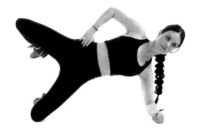

BANDED GLUTE BRIDGE *p. 285*
3 x 20 **

SIDE-LYING HIP RAISE *p. 279*
3 x 10-15 each side **

*   *Hold the contraction for about 0.5-1 seconds until you release the band and straighten your arms.*

**   *Hold the contraction for about 0.5-1 seconds until you lower your hips.*

Rest between supersets: 30-45 seconds.

 5 minutes   COOL-DOWN

Repeat the cool-down from Monday: Full Body 1, *pp. 48–51.*

SATURDAY – ACTIVE REST DAY

See "Tuesday – Active Rest Day" of this week, *pp. 103–105* or "Tuesday – Active Rest Day" from Week 5, *pp. 88–91.*

SUNDAY – REST DAY

Now you can finally rest and review the past week:

- How were your training and nutrition so far?

- What is the greatest achievement you've had?

In the following table, you can continue to keep track of your food and fluid intake. Note how many servings of protein, carbohydrates, and fats you have eaten. Use the required number of portions per day from the previous week.

Track the daily intake of protein, carbs, fats, vegetables, and the amount of water intake.

	Protein*	Carbs*	Fats*	Veggies*	Water*
Required portions per day					
Monday					
Tuesday					
Wednesday					
Thursday					
Friday					
Saturday					
Sunday					

*Please enter your own quantity.

Next week we will discuss an important topic: emotions and food. Stay tuned!

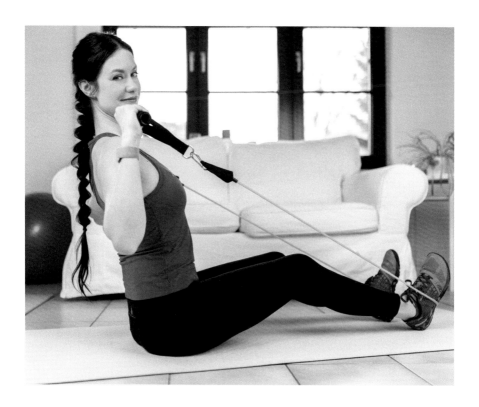

4.2.3 WEEK 7

This week's workouts are the same as in Week 5, but we will adjust the number of repetitions in each exercise. Notice how the number of repetitions varies depending on what type of equipment or resistance you use: a resistance band, dumbbells, or another kind of weight where you can change the load or resistance.

The last repetition of each set should be challenging but doable. At the same time, the execution form should always remain correct.

NUTRITION

Many trainers and athletes often consider food merely as fuel for our bodies. Just like cars' tanks that you fill with gasoline, you "fill up" your body with various nutrients (proteins, carbohydrates, fats, vitamins, and minerals) to have enough energy for physical or athletic performance. It is often said that food doesn't have to taste good. Just think of it as a source of energy.

However, the reality is quite different. Yes, food is our energy source, but it is also so much more than that. Food is a significant part of our lives. Every culture and religion has certain traditions associated with certain dishes and food culture. Every family also has its own traditions and preferences. When we meet with friends, go to birthdays and celebrations, or spend a relaxing evening at home, this is all connected with food in a certain way. And we can't simply exclude it from our lives because we also associate our feelings and emotions with it.

Imagine the following situation:

You have decided to lose a few pounds. Then you start a strict diet and have a very strong idea of what you can and cannot eat. Now you are invited to your relatives' birthday party. The table is all set, and there's a cake, too.

You told yourself you can't eat something like that, but the cake looks so delicious, and everyone enjoys it and tells you to have a piece too.

After all, there's no harm in it. You give in and eat a small piece, which tastes so good! But what happens next?

If you continue to spend your day normally and eat mindfully during your next meals, perhaps reducing the portions of carbs and fats you eat, everything will be fine. However, it is not uncommon to feel real guilt instead because you didn't follow through with your diet and gave in. In some cases, people completely lose control and start to eat large amounts of food. Others tend to do the opposite and punish themselves with food deprivation afterward.

Another possible scenario would be that you start worrying so much about the extra calories that you will hardly eat anything at this event because it doesn't fit your idea of a "healthy" diet, or you can't weigh the food down to the gram. As a result, you exclude yourself from the festivities and can't really enjoy the time with your family.

These are just a few real-life examples. However, the whole conversation about this topic is very complex, and one could write the entire book just about it. The key takeaway is that emotions and food are inseparable because *food is much more than just an energy source.*

Your task for this week is to discover your emotions in relation to food and try to understand them. For this, you can choose one to three days of the week (e.g., two weekdays and one weekend day) and keep a kind of diary in which you write down when and what you ate, as well as what you did, thought, or felt during, shortly before, or shortly after the meal.

For now, it's just about documenting. We will analyze it at the end of the week.

Here is a sample template for you:

Time	What did you eat?	What were you doing, feeling, or thinking?
9:30 p.m.	One chocolate bar	I was alone in the living room and suddenly started craving chocolate.

MONDAY – FULL BODY 1

 WARM-UP (NO EQUIPMENT NEEDED) 5 minutes

Repeat the warm-up from Monday: Full Body 1, *pp. 44–45.*

 WORKOUT approx. 30-35 minutes

SUPERSET 1:

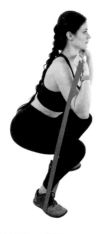 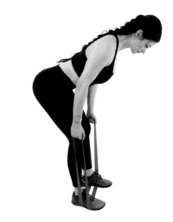

FRONT SQUAT *p. 274*　　　ROMANIAN DEADLIFT *p. 278*
4 x 15　　　　　　　　　　4 x 15

SUPERSET 2:

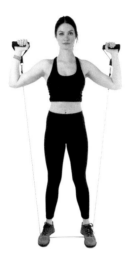

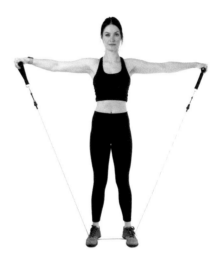

SHOULDER PRESS *p. 239*
4 x 15

LATERAL RAISE *p. 240*
4 x 15

SUPERSET 3:

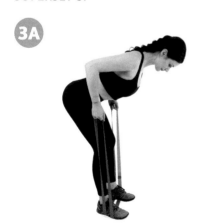

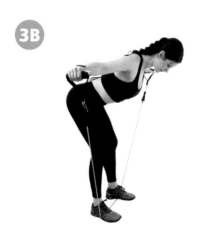

BENT-OVER ROW *p. 254*
4 x 15

BENT-OVER LATERAL RAISE *p. 241*
4 x 15

SUPERSET 4:

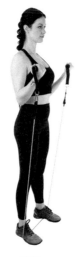

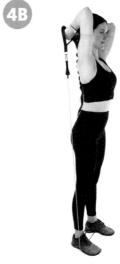

BICEPS CURL *p. 297*
3 x 15

OVERHEAD TRICEPS
EXTENSION *p. 301*
3 x 15

Rest between supersets: 30-45 seconds.

 ## COOL-DOWN

 5 minutes

Repeat the cool-down from Monday: Full Body 1, *pp. 48-50.*

TUESDAY - ACTIVE REST DAY

Choose one of the options:

• 20 minutes of light cardio exercise at a heart rate of 60%-70% of the HR max (see "Tuesday – Active Rest Day" from Week 5), *p. 88.*

• "Circuit 1" from Week 5, *pp. 90-91.*

• "Circuit 2" from Week 6, *pp. 104-105.*

WEDNESDAY – FULL BODY 2

 5 minutes WARM-UP (NO EQUIPMENT NEEDED)

Repeat the warm-up from Monday: Full Body 1, *pp. 44–45.*

 approx. 30-35 minutes WORKOUT

SUPERSET 1:

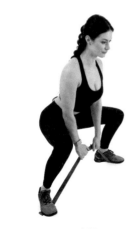

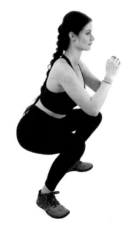

SUMO SQUAT *p. 282*
4 x 15

JUMP SQUAT *p. 268*
4 x 10-12

SUPERSET 2:

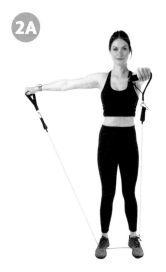

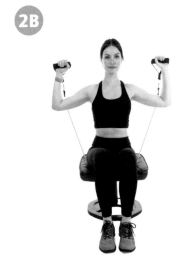

ALTERNATING FRONT AND
LATERAL RAISE *p. 234*
4 x 14

SHOULDER PRESS *p. 239*
4 x 15

SUPERSET 3:

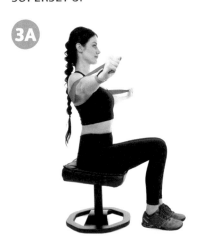

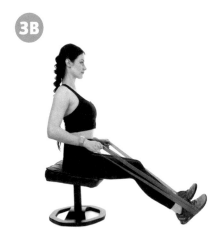

SEATED FLY *p. 247*
4 x 15 *

SEATED ROW *p. 252*
4 x 15 **

SUPERSET 4:

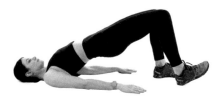

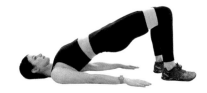

B-STANCE GLUTE BRIDGE *p. 284*
3 x 20 each side

BANDED GLUTE BRIDGE *p. 285*
3 x 20 * * *

*   *If the exercise is performed with dumbbells or weight, it should be performed while lying on the back.*

* *   *Hold the contraction for about 0.5-1 seconds until you release the band and straighten your arms.*

* * *   *Hold the contraction for about 0.5-1 seconds until you lower your hips.*

TIP

Position the resistance band around your knees if you need additional resistance for the "Glute Bridge" or "Hip Thrusts" exercises and their variations. If you are using dumbbells or another weight, place it on your hips.

Rest between supersets: 30-45 seconds.

 5 minutes   **COOL-DOWN**

Repeat the cool-down from Monday: Full Body 1, *pp. 48–50.*

THURSDAY – ACTIVE REST DAY

Choose one of the options:

- 20 minutes of light cardio exercise at a heart rate of 60%-70% of the HR_{max} (see "Tuesday – Active Rest Day" from Week 5), *p. 88.*

- "Circuit 1" from Week 5, *pp. 90–91.*

- "Circuit 2" from Week 6, *pp. 104–105.*

FRIDAY – FULL BODY 3

 WARM-UP (NO EQUIPMENT NEEDED)   **5 minutes**

Repeat the warm-up from Monday: Full Body 1, *pp. 44–45.*

 WORKOUT   **approx. 30-35 minutes**

SUPERSET 1:

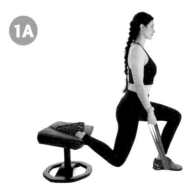

BULGARIAN SPLIT SQUAT *p. 266*
4 x 15 each side

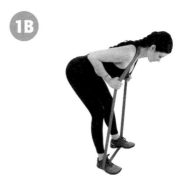

GOOD MORNING *p. 295*
4 x 15

SUPERSET 2:

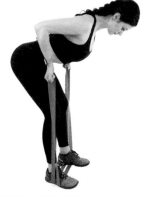

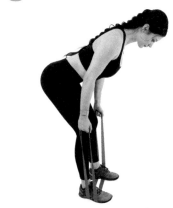

BENT-OVER ROW WITH SUPINATED GRIP *p. 255*
4 x 15

ROMANIAN DEADLIFT *p. 278*
4 x 15

SUPERSET 3:

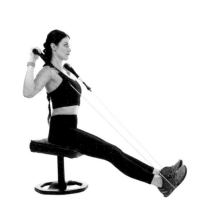

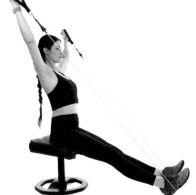

SEATED W ROW *p. 242*
4 x 15 *

SEATED Y RAISE *p. 244*
4 x 5-8 *

SUPERSET 4:

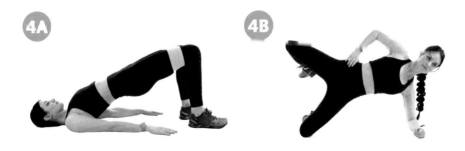

BANDED GLUTE BRIDGE *p. 285*
3 x 20-25 **

SIDE-LYING HIP RAISE *p. 279*
3 x 10-15 each side **

*   *Hold the contraction for about 0.5-1 seconds until you release the band and straighten your arms.*

**   *Hold the contraction for about 0.5-1 seconds until you lower your hips.*

Rest between supersets: 30-45 seconds.

 COOL-DOWN

 5 minutes

Repeat the cool-down from Monday: Full Body 1, *pp. 48–50.*

SATURDAY – ACTIVE REST DAY

Choose one of the options:

- 20 minutes of light cardio exercise at a heart rate of 60-70% of the HR_{max} (see "Tuesday - Active Rest Day" from Week 5), *p. 88.*

- "Circuit 1" from Week 5, *pp. 90–91.*

- "Circuit 2" from Week 6, *pp. 104–105.*

SUNDAY - REST DAY

Now you can finally rest and review the past week:

- Let's start with your journal about your emotions. Do you notice a trend, or do you see something that stands out?

- Separately, how were your training and nutrition so far?

- What is the greatest achievement you've had?

In the following table, you can continue to keep track of your nutrition.

Track the daily intake of protein, carbs, fats, vegetables, and the amount of water intake.

	Protein*	Carbs*	Fats*	Veggies*	Water*
Required portions per day					
Monday					
Tuesday					
Wednesday					
Thursday					
Friday					
Saturday					
Sunday					

*Please enter your own quantity

Next week we will continue talking about emotions, as well as stress and cravings.

4.2.4 WEEK 8

This week's workouts are the same as in Week 6, but we will adjust the number of repetitions in each exercise. The last repetition of each set should be challenging but doable. At the same time, the execution form should always remain technically correct.

This week is also the last week of Phase 2, so try to get everything out of it and do your best! Next week we will start training the upper and lower body separately.

NUTRITION

Last week we discussed the connection between emotions and food, and you probably discovered a lot about yourself. This week we'll talk about cravings or the need to eat something immediately. Many people usually crave something sweet – and other types of food – and often experience these feelings in the evening [Meule, 2020].

Today I will introduce you to a technique to help you understand your cravings and how to deal with them better.

HALT Technique

H – Hungry

A – Angry

L – Lonely

T – Tired

If you suddenly get a craving, take a minute and ask yourself if perhaps you haven't eaten for a while and are just hungry, or had poor quality sleep, or just not enough sleep. Or maybe you are upset or stressed about something, tired, lonely, or bored?

Now try to use this method every day until Thursday of this week. For now, it's all about observing, discovering, and interpreting your body's cues correctly.

MONDAY – FULL BODY 1

 5 minutes   WARM-UP (NO EQUIPMENT NEEDED)

Repeat the warm-up from Monday: Full Body 1, *pp. 44–45.*

 approx. 30-35 minutes   WORKOUT

SUPERSET 1:

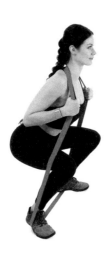

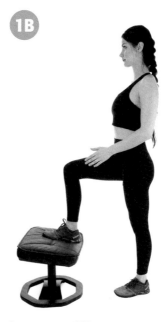

SQUAT *p. 271*
4 x 15

STEP-UP *p. 281*
4 x 15 each side

SUPERSET 2:

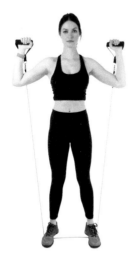

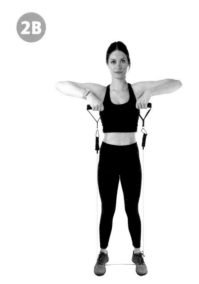

SHOULDER PRESS *p. 239*
4 x 15

UPRIGHT ROW *p. 236*
4 x 15

SUPERSET 3:

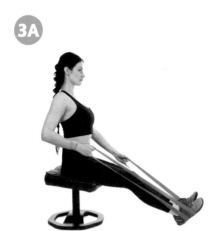

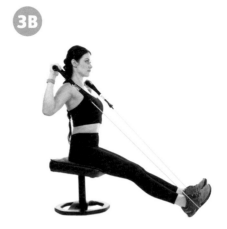

SINGLE-ARM ROW *p. 250*
4 x 15 each side

SEATED W ROW *p. 242*
4 x 15

SUPERSET 4:

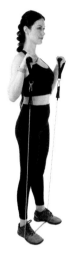

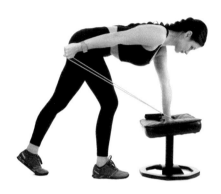

BICEPS CURL WITH PRONATED GRIP *p. 299*
3 x 15

TRICEPS KICKBACK *p. 302*
3 x 15 each side

Rest between supersets: 30-45 seconds.

 5 minutes COOL-DOWN

Repeat the cool-down from Monday: Full Body 1, *pp. 48–50.*

TUESDAY – ACTIVE REST DAY

Choose one of the options:

- 20 minutes of light cardio exercise at a heart rate of 60%-70% of the HR_{max} (see "Tuesday - Active Rest Day" from Week 5), *p. 88.*

- "Circuit 1" from Week 5, *pp. 90–91.*

- "Circuit 2" from Week 6, *pp. 104–105.*

WEDNESDAY – FULL BODY 2

 WARM-UP (NO EQUIPMENT NEEDED) **5 minutes**

Repeat the warm-up from Monday: Full Body 1, *pp. 44–45.*

 WORKOUT **approx. 30-35 minutes**

SUPERSET 1:

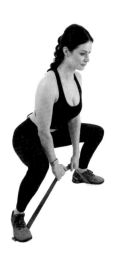

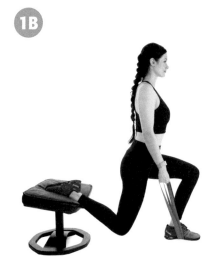

SUMO SQUAT *p. 282*
4 x 15

BULGARIAN SPLIT SQUAT *p. 266*
4 x 12 each side

SUPERSET 2:

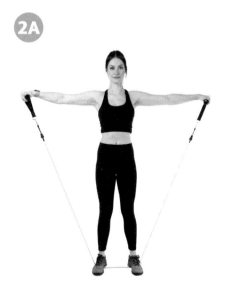

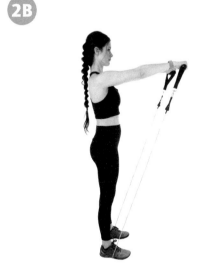

LATERAL RAISE *p. 240*
4 x 15

FRONT RAISE *p. 237*
4 x 12

SUPERSET 3:

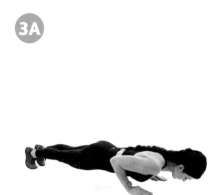

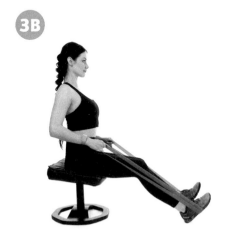

NARROW PUSH-UP *p. 303*
4 x 12

SEATED ROW *p. 252*
4 x 15 *

SUPERSET 4:

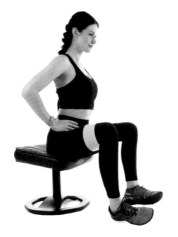

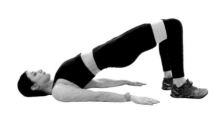

THREE-WAY SEATED BANDED HIP ABDUCTION (STRAIGHT UP/LEANING BACK/LEANING FORWARD) *p. 288*
3 x 20/20/20

BANDED GLUTE BRIDGE *p. 285*
3 x 20 **

* Hold the contraction for about 0.5-1 seconds until you release the band and straighten your arms.

** Hold the contraction for about 0.5-1 seconds until you lower your hips.

Rest between supersets: 30-45 seconds.

 COOL-DOWN

 5 minutes

Repeat the cool-down from Monday: Full Body 1, *pp. 48-50.*

NUTRITION (HALT TECHNIQUE)

What have you been able to discover so far?

From now on, we can go one step further. When you start craving something, ask yourself whether you're hungry, stressed, lonely, bored, or tired. If you are actually hungry, simply eat a balanced meal. (See the following Note.)

However, if it's not about hunger as such, just sit on your feelings for five minutes. Notice these feelings, your thoughts at that moment, and your physical discomfort.

After five minutes, you're free to do whatever you want. You can eat what you've been dying to eat . . . or not: it's up to you.

You may wonder what the point of this is. Being mindful of yourself and being able to notice your body cues is crucial. Even though this method may not seem noteworthy to you, it can help you in the long run by giving you control over your feelings and gaining more self-confidence. And, in the long run, even the smallest changes will lead to a big one.

NOTE

If your goal is to lose weight, you will feel hungry at some point during your dietary change. This is a normal reaction of your body, which is inevitable because your body does not know about your diet. It only knows that you are eating less food and your energy depots are losing fat. Your body reacts this way so you don't starve.

This hormonal response is a protective mechanism of your body. The more fat you lose, the more hunger you will feel. What you can do is increase your meal size by, for example, eating more vegetables or foods with a lower caloric density (i.e., the number of calories per 100 g). Sometimes, however, depending on how much weight you want to lose, you just can't avoid the hunger sensation, and you have to learn to tolerate a light hunger feeling.

THURSDAY – ACTIVE REST DAY

Choose one of the options:

- 20 minutes of light cardio exercise at a heart rate of 60-70% of the HR_{max} (see "Tuesday – Active Rest Day" from Week 5), *p. 88.*

- "Circuit 1" from Week 5, *pp. 90–91.*

- "Circuit 2" from Week 6, *pp. 104–105.*

FRIDAY – FULL BODY 3

 ## WARM-UP (NO EQUIPMENT NEEDED)   **5 minutes**

Repeat the warm-up from Monday: Full Body 1, *pp. 44–45.*

 ## WORKOUT   **approx. 30-35 minutes**

SUPERSET 1:

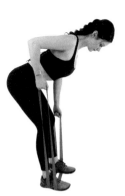

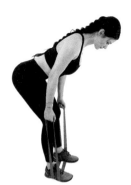

BENT-OVER SINGLE-ARM ROW *p. 253*
4 x 15 each side

ROMANIAN DEADLIFT *p. 278*
4 x 15

134

SUPERSET 2:

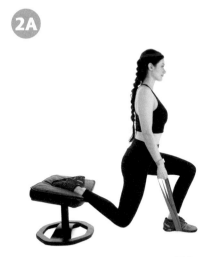

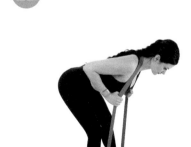

BULGARIAN SPLIT SQUAT *p. 266*
4 x 15 each side

GOOD MORNING *p. 295*
4 x 15

SUPERSET 3:

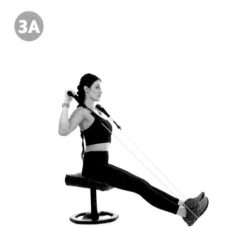

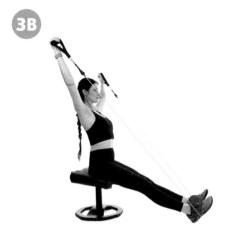

SEATED W ROW *p. 242*
4 x 15 *

SEATED Y RAISE *p. 244*
4 x 8 *

SUPERSET 4:

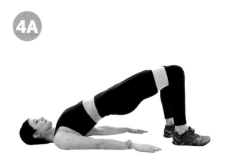

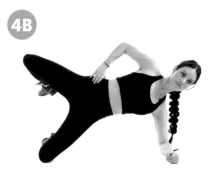

BANDED GLUTE BRIDGE *p. 285*
3 x 20**

SIDE-LYING HIP RAISE *p. 279*
3 x 10-15 each side **

* *Hold the contraction for about 0.5-1 seconds until you release the band and straighten your arms.*

** *Hold the contraction for about 0.5-1 seconds until you lower your hips.*

Rest between supersets: 30-45 seconds.

COOL-DOWN

 5 minutes

Repeat the cool-down from Monday: Full Body 1, *pp. 48–50.*

SATURDAY – ACTIVE REST DAY

Choose one of the options:

- 20 minutes of light cardio exercise at a heart rate of 60%-70% of the HR_{max} (see "Tuesday – Active Rest Day" from Week 5), *p. 88.*

- "Circuit 1" from Week 5, *pp. 90–91.*

- "Circuit 2" from Week 6, *pp. 104–105.*

SUNDAY – REST DAY

Now you can finally rest and review the past week:

- What did you learn about yourself this week?

- How were your training and nutrition?

- What is the greatest achievement you've had?

In the following table, you can continue to keep track of your nutrition. Note how many servings of protein, carbohydrates, and fats you have eaten. Use the required number of portions per day from the previous week.

Track the daily intake of protein, carbs, fats, vegetables, and the amount of water intake.

	Protein*	Carbs*	Fats*	Veggies*	Water*
Required portions per day					
Monday					
Tuesday					
Wednesday					
Thursday					
Friday					
Saturday					
Sunday					

*Please enter your own quantity

Tomorrow the third training phase starts. Therefore, I would like to remind you that you can do each training phase longer than four weeks. You can repeat Phases 1 and 2 one more time, or each phase twice, or you can do each week twice before moving on to the next training session. The most important thing is to adjust your bands' resistance or weight used each week.

137

Tomorrow you should also check your progress: Weight, progress photos, and body measurements. If you are not concerned with your appearance, write down how you feel and if you think anything has changed.

- Maybe you feel stronger?

- Were you able to complete your workout despite your other responsibilities?

- Or, have you developed a new habit that brings you closer to your goal?

Next week will be all about your sleep.

4.3 Phase 3

Congratulations! You have completed the first two phases and created a good foundation. Now we will work even more precisely on your body and divide your training into lower- and upper-body sessions.

The goal of this phase is to focus more on specific muscle groups and eliminate possible weaknesses or imbalances if you have any.

As described in chapter 2, you will do four main training sessions in this training phase – two for the lower body and two for the upper body. When you train your lower body, you will also do abs exercises.

Furthermore, there are two additional workouts per week: one workout for your glutes and one for your shoulders. These are optional; you can do just one of the workouts or both. For better results, I recommend doing all six suggested weekly workouts. However, if it's too much for you, feel free to work out only five times per week (twice upper body, twice lower body, and either shoulder or glutes) or four times per week (twice upper body, twice lower body).

If you choose the latter option, I recommend staying active on two of three non-training days. As in Phase 2, there are several options for doing so:

- 20 minutes of light cardio exercise at a heart rate of 60%-70% of the HR_{max} (see "Tuesday – Active Rest Day" from Week 5), *p. 88.*

- "Circuit 1" from Week 5, *pp. 90–91.*

- "Circuit 2" from Week 6, *pp. 104–105.*

Your weekly schedule will look like this:

MONDAY	Lower Body 1 + Abs
TUESDAY	Upper Body 1
WEDNESDAY	Shoulders or alternatively Active Rest Day
THURSDAY	Lower Body 2 + Abs
FRIDAY	Upper Body 2
SATURDAY	Glutes or alternatively Active Rest Day
SUNDAY	Rest Day

NOTE

You don't necessarily have to start every Monday. You can choose the day that suits you best. However, do not change the order of the workouts.

4.3.1 WEEK 9

Since you'll be training your upper and lower body separately starting this week, your warm-up and cool-down routines will be adjusted accordingly. If you're training your shoulders, your warm-up and cool-down will be the same as for your upper body. And if you are training your glutes, we will repeat your warm-up and cool-down from the lower body workout.

For this and the remaining weeks, try to perform all movements in a controlled and slow manner. Unless otherwise instructed, choose your resistance (band or weight) so that you can still complete the last repetition with a good execution form. However, if you had to do one to two more repetitions with that resistance, you would not be physically able to.

Question:

I don't want to look like a man. Should I then just train the lower body and abs?

Answer:

Don't worry about it. You will not look like a man if you train your upper body separately. This is simply impossible due to the hormonal differences between men and women! Also, you won't build muscle mass as quickly, and therefore you'll be able to control your body shape very well.

By training your upper body, you will develop a toned and nicer back and arms. Your posture will improve, and you will generally highlight your feminine physique positively.

If you already have a very athletic physique with little body fat and don't want your arms to get any bigger, simply choose a lighter resistance when working out. However, do not entirely stop training these muscle groups.

PROGRESS MONITORING AND NUTRITION

Before we start the training week, we want to recheck your progress. As described before the first training week, you can weigh yourself, take your body measurements, and progress photos. Do this in the morning directly after getting up and after you have been to the bathroom but before eating or drinking anything.

Now analyze your results. Refer again to section 4.2.1 (Week 5) and section 5.1. If everything is going according to your plan, do not change anything for now. Just continue your diet exactly as before, and do not change your portion sizes.

However, if things are not going as planned, check how you can optimize your diet. For this, you can have a look at chapter 3. Regularly ask yourself if there is anything you can do better in your nutrition and then try to implement it step by step.

TIP

Try to eat enough carbohydrates before and after training (at least one cupped hand). For the remaining meals, you can make the portions a little smaller. Keep in mind the total amount of carbs for the day.

RECOVERY

The last four weeks will be even more intense than the previous ones since you will be doing more training sessions. Recovery will become even more of a priority.

This week we will first discuss your sleep. Everyone knows how important sleep is, but at the same time, it is still too often underestimated and neglected. People always seek the right tool or the best supplement to improve their performance or accelerate their progress, yet research shows that longer sleep alone positively impacts your athletic performance (Kirschen et al., 2020), your body composition, and your fat loss (Jabekk et al., 2020). Implementing a nap can also be a good strategy if you had a bad night.

TIPS FOR IMPROVING YOUR SLEEP

These tips will help you fall asleep faster as well as improve the quality of your sleep (Watson, 2017):

- Always go to bed at the same time and try to get up at about the same time each day.

- Keep a diary to understand how long you sleep. Ideally, you can do this with the help of a smartwatch or fitness tracker. Over time, you can figure out how long you should rest so you feel refreshed and energized. Most people need between seven and eight hours of sleep at night.

- Your bedroom should be dark and cool.

- The bedroom and your bed should only be used for sleep and sex.

- Smartphone and screen use can suppress the natural production of the sleep hormone melatonin. Therefore, try not to use your phone and turn off the TV for about an hour or at least 30 minutes before bed. Alternatively, you can wear special glasses in the evening that block the "blue light" of the screens.

- Caffeine or caffeinated beverages are best consumed only in the morning.

As with the other tips about your diet or exercise, try not to implement them all at once. Choose one to three tips that you find exciting and implement them consistently over two to three weeks before you start making the next changes.

MONDAY – LOWER BODY 1 + ABS

 5 minutes **WARM-UP (NO EQUIPMENT NEEDED)**

If you're training with resistance bands only, do the following warm-up routine:

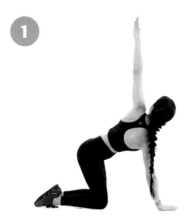

THREAD THE NEEDLE * *p. 312*
2 each side

WIDE KNEE CHILD POSE ** *p. 310*
2-3 reps

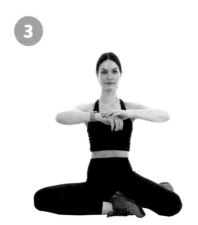

HIP AND KNEE MOBILIZATION *p. 308*
2 each side

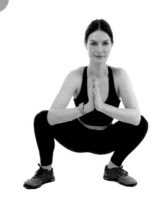

DEEP SQUAT WITH ANKLE ROCKING
p. 309
30 seconds

*   *The spine is almost always loaded, so we should mobilize it even during lower body training. This way, we ensure that the vertebrae are mobilized and not misaligned when the spine is loaded.*

**   *Although the exercise stretches the chest and back muscles to some degree, this is also very useful in lower body training. Often these muscles are shortened by everyday life due to frequent sitting, which directly affects our posture and, therefore, our spine.*

If you train with dumbbells or heavy weights, I recommend you extend your warm-up a bit. For example, you can add the following exercises to the ones listed above:

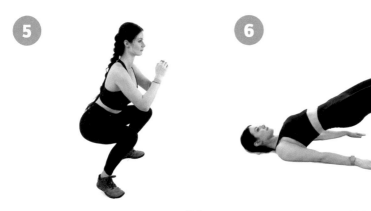

5

6

BODY WEIGHT DEEP SQUAT *p. 316*
10 reps

GLUTE BRIDGE * *p. 305*
10 reps

*Focus on contracting your glutes

approx. 35-40 minutes

WORKOUT

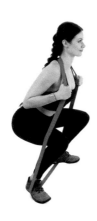

SQUAT *p. 271*
3 x 15

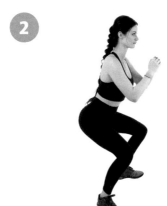

PULSE SQUAT *p. 277*
2 x 15

3

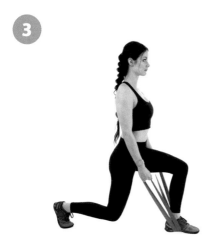

REVERSE LUNGE *p. 265*
4 x 15 each side

4

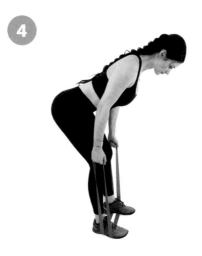

ROMANIAN DEADLIFT * *p. 278*
4 x 15

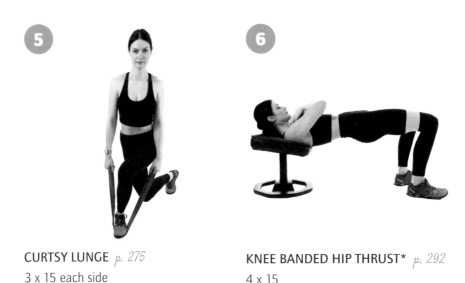

CURTSY LUNGE *p. 275*
3 x 15 each side

KNEE BANDED HIP THRUST* *p. 292*
4 x 15

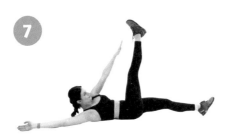

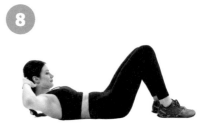

JACKKNIFE CROSSOVER *p. 259*
3 x 15 each side

CRUNCH *p. 257*
2 x AMRAP**

*   *Slowly lower the upper body in exercise 4 or the hips in exercise 6 (3-4 seconds) and quickly straighten up or lift the pelvis (one second).*

**   *Do as many repetitions as you can. Make sure your belly stays flat and doesn't bulge or dome. If you can't hold the tension and your abdomen starts bulging, stop the exercise or take a break.*

Rest between sets: 30-60 seconds. You should feel rested before the next set but not completely relaxed.

5 minutes COOL-DOWN

The cool-down after the lower body workout is from Week 1, Monday – Full Body 1, but you will only partially adopt it. Hold each position for a few seconds (10-30 seconds, or as long as it's comfortable for you), feel the stretch in the muscles, and breathe deeply.

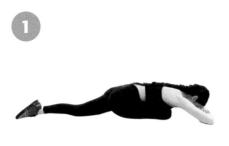

PIGEON TO HALF PIGEON POSE TO SINGLE-LEG FORWARD BEND POSE ONE SIDE *p. 326*

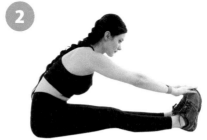

SEATED FORWARD BEND *p. 321*

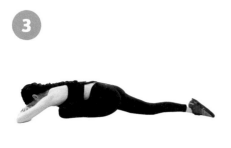

Repeat 1 for the opposite side

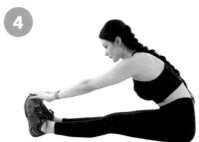

Repeat 2

147

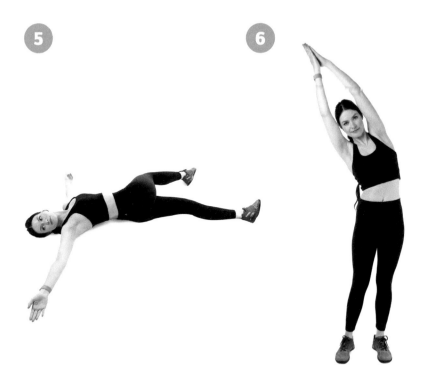

5

6

SUPINE SPINAL TWIST *p. 323*

STANDING SIDE BEND *p. 315*
Hold 1-2 seconds per side

TUESDAY – UPPER BODY 1

 5 minutes   WARM-UP (NO EQUIPMENT NEEDED)

If you're training with resistance bands only, do the following warm-up routine:

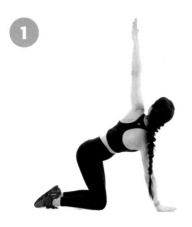

THREAD THE NEEDLE *p. 312*
2 each side

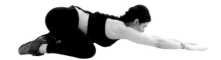

CHILD POSE *p. 322*
Hold the stretch in each repetition for at least 1-2 seconds

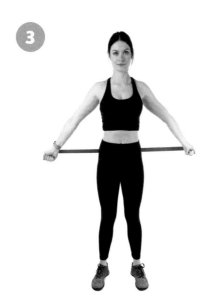

BANDED SHOULDER CIRCLES *p. 313*
2 in each direction

If you train with dumbbells or heavy weights, I recommend you extend your warm-up a bit. For example, you can add the following exercises to the ones listed before:

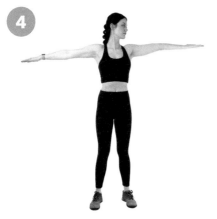

STRAIGHT-ARM SHOULDER ROTATION *p. 314*

5 reps each side

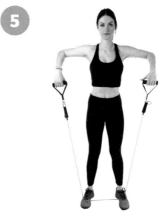

CUBAN PRESS WITH VERY LIGHT WEIGHTS *p. 306*

8 reps

 WORKOUT

 approx. 35-40 minutes

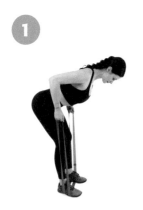

BENT-OVER ROW * *p. 254*

3 x 15

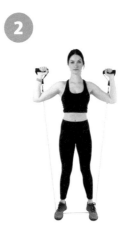

SHOULDER PRESS *p. 239*

3 x 15

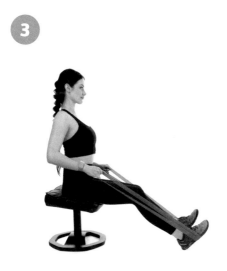

SEATED ROW * *p. 252*
3 x 12

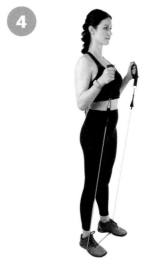

HAMMER CURL * *p. 298*
3 x 12

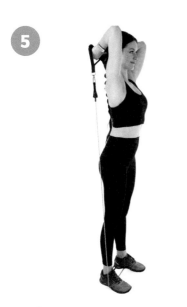

**OVERHEAD TRICEPS
EXTENSION *** *p. 301*
3 x 12

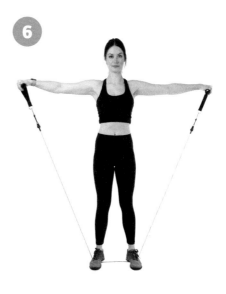

LATERAL RAISE *p. 240*
3 x 12

7

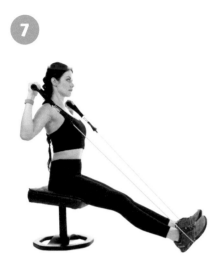

**SEATED W ROW ** *p. 242*
2 x 10-15

*   *In the end position, when your muscles are contracted, hold the tension for 0.5-1 second before slowly lowering your arms.*

**   *Focus on the contracting muscles and make the movement slow and controlled. During the exercise, it is essential that you feel the back of your shoulders and that your shoulders and shoulder blades are not lifted up when pulling the band. If the band you use is too challenging, you can use a lighter weight instead, such as a water bottle or two books, and then perform the exercise bent over.*

Rest between sets: 30-60 seconds. You should feel rested before the next set but not completely relaxed.

5 minutes COOL-DOWN

The cool-down after the upper body workout will be different from the previous weeks. Hold each position for a few seconds (10-30 seconds or as long as you are comfortable), feel the stretch in the muscles, and breathe deeply.

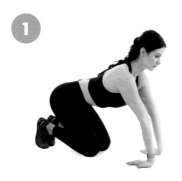

BICEPS AND FOREARM STRETCH *p. 319*

CHILD POSE *p. 322*

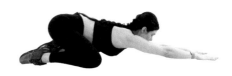

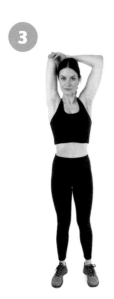

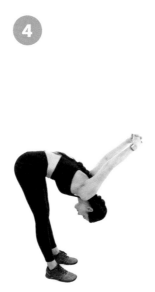

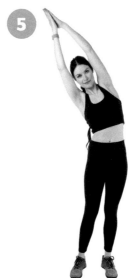

TRICEPS STRETCH
p. 327

STANDING FORWARD BEND WITH SHOULDER OPENER
p. 329

STANDING SIDE BEND
p. 315
Hold 1-2 seconds per side

WEDNESDAY – SHOULDERS OR ALTERNATIVELY ACTIVE REST DAY

If you prefer to take a break from training today, you can choose one of the following options:

- 20 minutes of light cardio exercise at a heart rate of 60%-70% of the HR$_{max}$ (see "Tuesday – Active Rest Day" from Week 5), *p. 88.*

- "Circuit 1" from Week 5, *pp. 90–91.*

- "Circuit 2" from Week 6, *pp. 104–105.*

Alternatively, you can train your shoulders today. You can find the workout next.

 ## WARM-UP (NO EQUIPMENT NEEDED) **5 minutes**

Repeat this week's warm-up from Tuesday - Upper Body 1, *pp. 149–150.*

 ## WORKOUT **approx. 25-30 minutes**

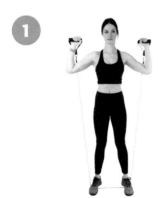

SHOULDER PRESS *p. 239*
4 x 15

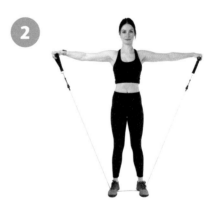

LATERAL RAISE *p. 240*
3 x 15

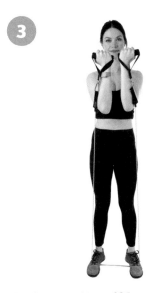

ARNOLD PRESS *p. 235*
4 x 12

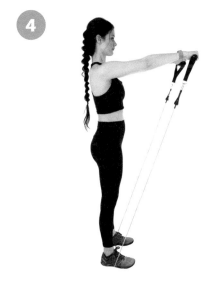

FRONT RAISE *p. 237*
3 x 12

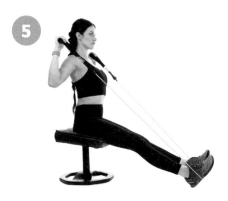

SEATED W ROW *p. 242*
4 x 12

Rest between sets: 30-45 seconds.

COOL-DOWN

 5 minutes

Hold each position for a few seconds (10-30 seconds or as long as you are comfortable), feel the stretch in the muscles, and breathe deeply.

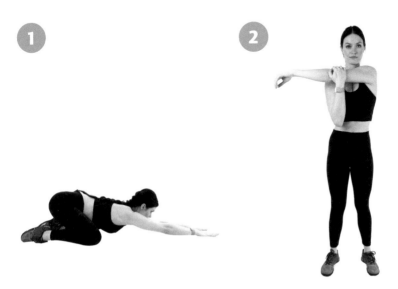

CHILD POSE *p. 322*

SIDE DELTOID STRETCH *p. 324*

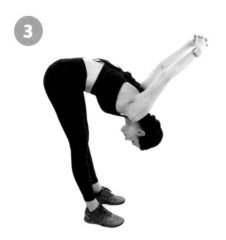

STANDING FORWARD BEND WITH SHOULDER OPENER *p. 329*

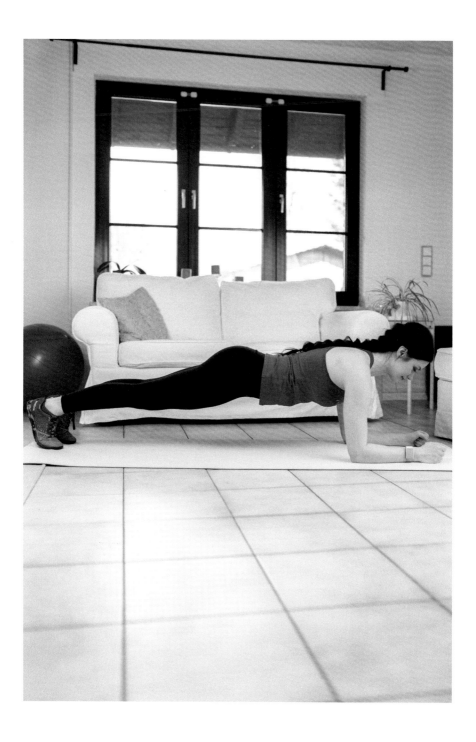

THURSDAY – LOWER BODY 2 + ABS

 ## WARM-UP (NO EQUIPMENT NEEDED)   **5 minutes**

Repeat this week's warm-up from Monday – Lower Body 1 + Abs, *pp. 143–144.*

 ## WORKOUT   **approx. 35-40 minutes**

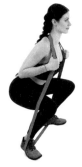

SQUAT *p. 271*
4 x 15

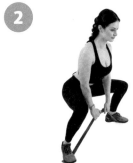

SUMO SQUAT *p. 282*
3 x 15

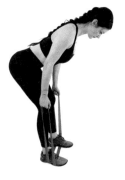

ROMANIAN DEADLIFT * *p. 278*
4 x 15

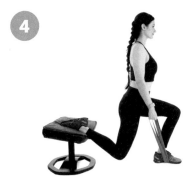

BULGARIAN SPLIT SQUAT *p. 266*
4 x 12 each side

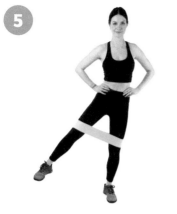

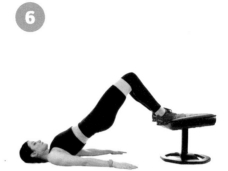

BANDED LEG ABDUCTION *p. 287*
3 x 12 each side

ELEVATED BANDED GLUTE BRIDGE *p. 286*
4 x 15

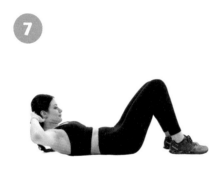

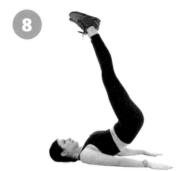

CRUNCH *p. 257*
3 x 15

REVERSE CRUNCH *p. 261*
3 x 15

* Slow lowering of the upper body (2-3 seconds) and quick straight up (one second).

Rest between sets: 30-60 seconds. You should feel rested before the next set but not completely relaxed.

 5 minutes   **COOL-DOWN**

Repeat this week's cool-down from Monday – Lower Body 1 + Abs, *pp. 147–148.*

FRIDAY – UPPER BODY 2

 WARM-UP (NO EQUIPMENT NEEDED) 5 minutes

Repeat this week's warm-up from Tuesday – Upper Body 1, *pp. 149–150.*

 WORKOUT approx. 30-35 minutes

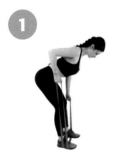

**BENT-OVER SINGLE-ARM
ROW *** *p. 253*
3 x 15 each side

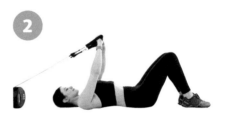

PULLOVER *p. 249*
3 x 15

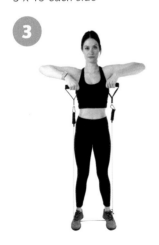

UPRIGHT ROW *p. 236*
3 x 15

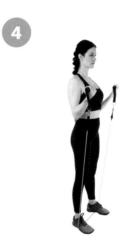

BICEPS CURL * *p. 297*
3 x 12

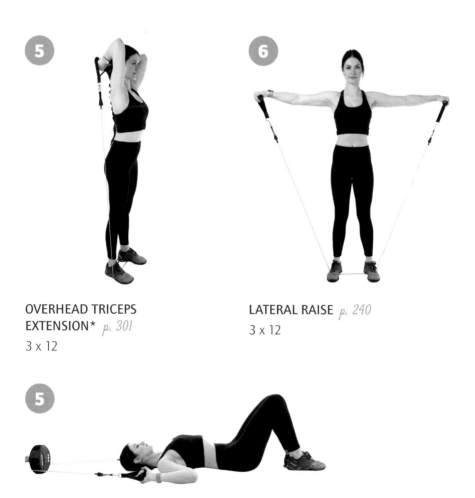

**OVERHEAD TRICEPS
EXTENSION*** *p. 301*
3 x 12

LATERAL RAISE *p. 240*
3 x 12

SUPINE LAT PULLDOWN *p. 251*
3 x 12

*   *In the end position, when your muscles are contracted, hold the tension for
0.5-1 second before slowly lowering your arms.*

Rest between sets: 30-60 seconds. You should feel rested before the next set but
not completely relaxed.

 5 minutes   COOL-DOWN

Repeat this week's cool-down from Tuesday – Upper Body 1, *p. 153.*

161

SATURDAY – GLUTES
OR ALTERNATIVELY ACTIVE REST DAY

If you prefer to take a break from training today, you can choose one of the following options:

- 20 minutes of light cardio exercise at a heart rate of 60%-70% of the HR_{max} (see "Tuesday – Active Rest Day" from Week 5), *p. 88.*

- "Circuit 1" from Week 5, *pp. 90–91.*

- "Circuit 2" from Week 6, *pp. 104–105.*

Alternatively, you can train your glutes today. You can find the workout next.

 ## WARM-UP (NO EQUIPMENT NEEDED)   **5 minutes**

Repeat this week's warm-up from Monday – Lower Body 1 + Abs, *pp. 143-144.*

 ## WORKOUT   **approx. 25-30 minutes**

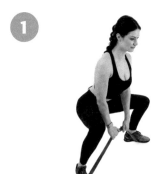

SUMO SQUAT *p. 282*
4 x 15

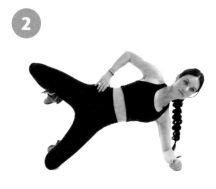

SIDE-LYING HIP RAISE *p. 279*
3 x 12 each side

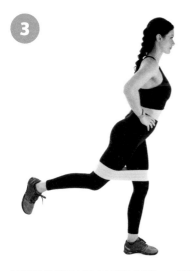

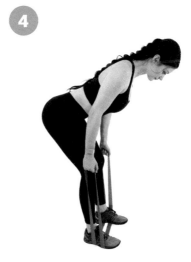

KNEE BANDED KICKBACK *p. 289*
3 x 12 each side

ROMANIAN DEADLIFT *p. 278*
4 x 15

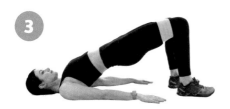

BANDED GLUTE BRIDGE *p. 285*
4 x 12

Try to perform all exercises a little slower. It is important that you feel the muscles well and perform the movement with a good execution form.

Rest between sets: 30-45 seconds.

 5 minutes   **COOL-DOWN**

Repeat this week's cool-down from Monday – Lower Body 1 + Abs, *pp. 147-148.*

SUNDAY – REST DAY

Now you can finally rest and review the past week:

- What did you learn about yourself this week?

- How were your training and nutrition?

- What is the greatest achievement you've had?

Continue to keep an eye on your nutrition and hydration.

Track the daily intake of protein, carbs, fats, vegetables, and the amount of water intake.

	Protein*	Carbs*	Fats*	Veggies*	Water*
Required portions per day					
Monday					
Tuesday					
Wednesday					
Thursday					
Friday					
Saturday					
Sunday					

*Please enter your own quantity

Next week, it's all about implementing all the previous tips consistently. Stick to the philosophy of doing "today a little bit better than yesterday."

In addition, you will get a few tips on reducing your stress which could boost your recovery.

4.3.2 WEEK 10

This and the remaining weeks are similar to Week 9, so you can continue to train only your lower and upper body or add extra workouts for your shoulders and glutes. It is up to you and your preference.

STRESS MANAGEMENT

Stress is inevitable in our lives. However, we need to learn how to deal with stressful situations to reduce the negative impact of stress. Sleep alone plays a major role in this process. It helps to reduce physical and also psychological stress, which, in turn, promotes regeneration.

Further stress management strategies can be chosen according to one's personal preferences and wishes (Kellmann et al., 2018).

Among others, the following options may be helpful:

- Relaxation techniques

- Yoga

- Meditation

- Walking in the fresh air

- A warm bath

- Massage

- Journaling.

And sometimes just talking to a good friend can really help!

Same as before, it doesn't matter which strategy you choose. Start slowly. Don't overwhelm and stress yourself even more by trying to implement everything at once!

MONDAY – LOWER BODY 1 + ABS

 WARM-UP (NO EQUIPMENT NEEDED) **5 minutes**

Repeat the warm-up from Monday – Lower Body 1 + Abs, *pp. 143-144.*

 WORKOUT **approx. 35-40 minutes**

1

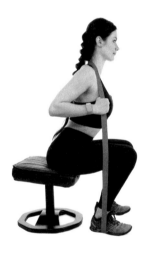

2

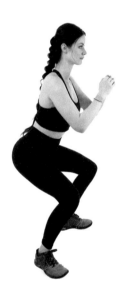

CHAIR OR BOX SQUAT * *p. 272*
4 x 15

PULSE SQUAT *p. 277*
2 x 15

3

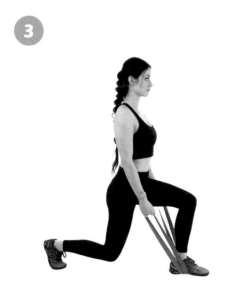

REVERSE LUNGE *p. 265*
4 x 15 each side

4

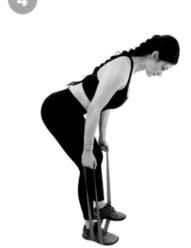

ROMANIAN DEADLIFT ** *p. 278*
4 x 15

5

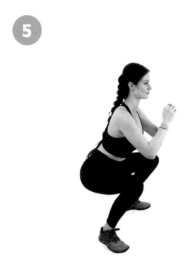

STATIC SQUAT HOLD *p. 280*
4 x 30 seconds

6

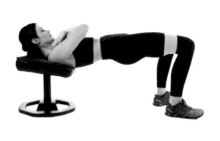

**KNEE BANDED HIP
THRUST** ** *p. 292*
4 x 20

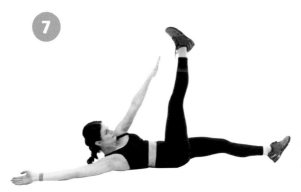

JACKKNIFE CROSSOVER
p. 259
3 x 15 each side

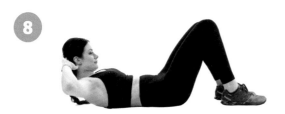

CRUNCH *p. 257*
2 x AMRAP***

*   *Get up from a chair.*

**   *Slowly lower the upper body in exercise 4 or the hips in exercise 6 (3-4 seconds) and quickly straighten up or lift the pelvis (one second).*

***   *Do as many repetitions as you can. Make sure your belly stays flat and doesn't bulge or dome. If you can't hold the tension and your abdomen starts bulging, stop the exercise or take a break.*

Rest between sets: 30-60 seconds. You should feel rested before the next set but not completely relaxed.

 COOL-DOWN **5 minutes**

Repeat the cool-down from Monday – Lower Body 1 + Abs, Week 9, *pp. 147-148.*

TUESDAY – UPPER BODY 1

 5 minutes   **WARM-UP (NO EQUIPMENT NEEDED)**

Repeat the warm-up from Tuesday – Upper Body 1, Week 9, *pp. 149–150.*

 approx. 35 minutes   **WORKOUT**

1

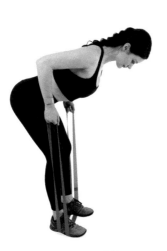

BENT-OVER ROW * *p. 254*
4 x 15

2

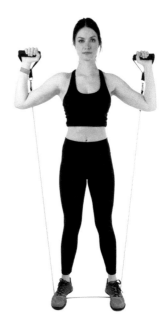

SHOULDER PRESS *p. 239*
4 x 15

169

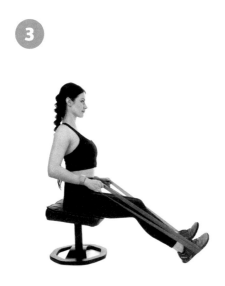

SEATED ROW * *p. 252*
4 x 15

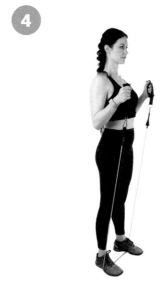

HAMMER CURL * *p. 298*
3 x 12

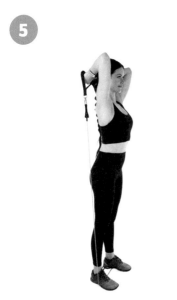

OVERHEAD TRICEPS EXTENSION* *p. 301*
3 x 12

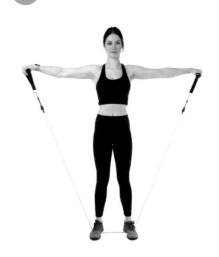

LATERAL RAISE *p. 240*
3 x 12

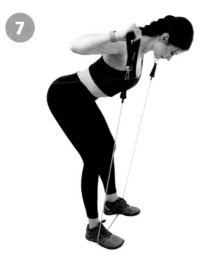

**BENT-OVER W ROW ** * * *p. 243*
3 x 10-15 * *

* In the end position, when your muscles are contracted, hold the tension for 0.5-1 second before slowly lowering your arms.

* * Focus on the contracting muscles and make the movement slow and controlled. During the exercise, it is essential that you feel the back of your shoulders and that your shoulders and shoulder blades are not lifted up when pulling the band. If the band you use is too challenging, you can use a lighter weight instead, such as a water bottle or two books.

Rest between sets: 30-60 seconds. You should feel rested before the next set but not completely relaxed.

 5 minutes COOL-DOWN

Repeat the cool-down from Tuesday – Upper Body 1, Week 9, *p. 153.*

WEDNESDAY – SHOULDERS
OR ALTERNATIVELY ACTIVE REST DAY 2

If you prefer to take a break from training today, you can choose one of the following options:

- 20 minutes of light cardio exercise at a heart rate of 60%-70% of the HR_{max} (see "Tuesday – Active Rest Day" from Week 5), *p. 88.*

- "Circuit 1" from Week 5, *pp. 90–91.*

- "Circuit 2" from Week 6, *pp. 104–105.*

Alternatively, you can train your shoulders today. You can find the workout next.

 ## WARM-UP (NO EQUIPMENT NEEDED) **5 minutes**

Repeat this week's warm-up from Tuesday – Upper Body 1, *pp. 149–150.*

 ## WORKOUT **approx. 25-30 minutes**

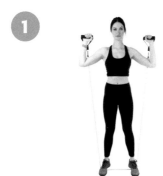

SHOULDER PRESS *p. 239*
4 x 15

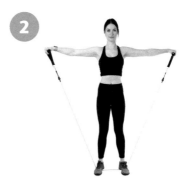

LATERAL RAISE *p. 240*
3 x 15

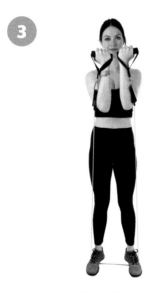

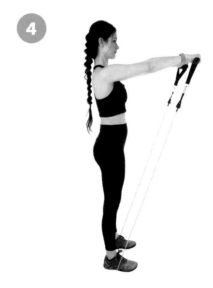

ARNOLD PRESS *p. 235*
4 x 15

FRONT RAISE *p. 237*
3 x 12

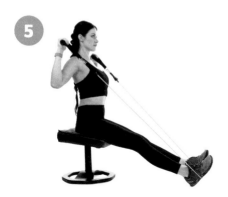

SEATED W ROW *p. 242*
4 x 12

Rest between sets: 30-45 seconds.

 5 minutes

COOL-DOWN

Repeat the cool-down from Wednesday – Shoulders, Week 9, *p. 156.*

THURSDAY – LOWER BODY 2 + ABS

 WARM-UP (NO EQUIPMENT NEEDED) **5 minutes**

Repeat the warm-up from Monday – Lower Body 1 + Abs, Week 9, *pp. 143–144.*

 WORKOUT **approx. 35-40 minutes**

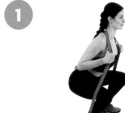

SQUAT *p. 271*
4 x 15

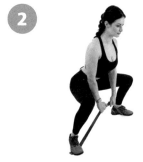

SUMO SQUAT *p. 282*
3 x 15

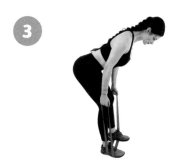

ROMANIAN DEADLIFT * *p. 278*
4 x 15

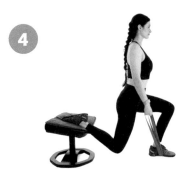

BULGARIAN SPLIT SQUAT *p. 266*
4 x 15 each side

174

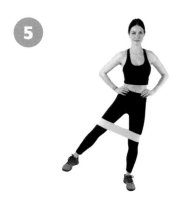

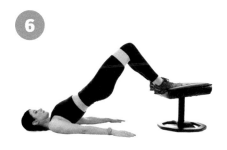

BANDED LEG ABDUCTION *p. 287*

3 x 15 each side

ELEVATED BANDED GLUTE BRIDGE *p. 286*

4 x 15

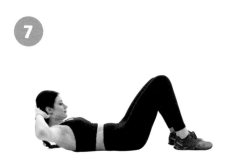

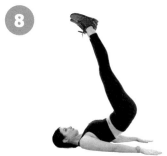

CRUNCH *p. 257*

3 x 15

REVERSE CRUNCH *p. 261*

3 x 15

* *Slow lowering of the upper body (2-3 seconds) and quick straight up (1 second).*

Rest between sets: 30-60 seconds. You should feel rested before the next set but not completely relaxed.

 5 minutes   **COOL-DOWN**

Repeat the cool-down from Monday – Lower Body 1 + Abs, Week 9, *pp. 147-148.*

FRIDAY – UPPER BODY 2

 WARM-UP (NO EQUIPMENT NEEDED) **5 minutes**

Repeat the warm-up from Tuesday – Upper Body 1, Week 9, *pp. 149–150.*

 WORKOUT **approx. 30-35 minutes**

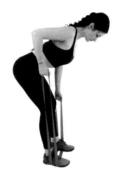

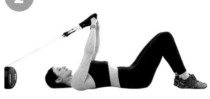

BENT-OVER SINGLE-ARM ROW * *p. 253*
4 x 15 each side

PULLOVER *p. 249*
4 x 15

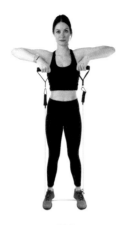

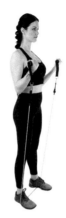

UPRIGHT ROW *p. 236*
4 x 15

BICEPS CURL * *p. 297*
3 x 15

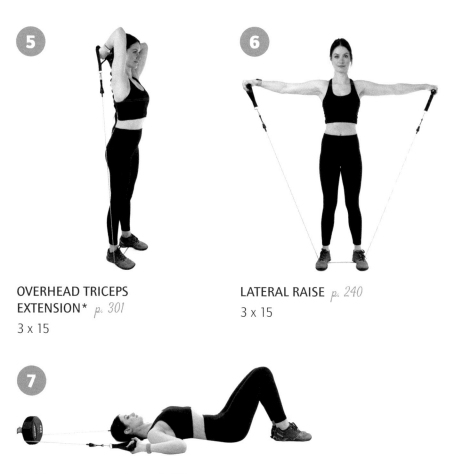

OVERHEAD TRICEPS EXTENSION* *p. 301*
3 x 15

LATERAL RAISE *p. 240*
3 x 15

SUPINE LAT PULLDOWN *S. 251*
4 x 15

*   *In the end position, when your muscles are contracted, hold the tension for 0.5-1 second before slowly lowering your arms.*

Rest between sets: 30-60 seconds. You should feel rested before the next set but not completely relaxed.

 5 minutes

COOL-DOWN

Repeat the cool-down from Tuesday – Upper Body 1, Week 9, *p. 153.*

SATURDAY – GLUTES
OR ALTERNATIVELY ACTIVE REST DAY

If you prefer to take a break from training today, you can choose one of the following options:

- 20 minutes of light cardio exercise at a heart rate of 60%-70% of the HR_{max} (see "Tuesday - Active Rest Day" from Week 5), *p. 88.*

- "Circuit 1" from Week 5, *pp. 90–91.*

- "Circuit 2" from Week 6, *pp. 104–105.*

Alternatively, you can train your glutes today. You can find the workout next.

 ## WARM-UP (NO EQUIPMENT NEEDED) **5 minutes**

Repeat the warm-up from Monday – Lower Body 1 + Abs, Week 9, *pp. 143-144.*

 ## WORKOUT **approx. 25-30 minutes**

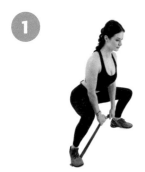

SUMO SQUAT *p. 282*
4 x 15

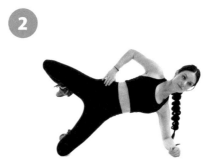

SIDE-LYING HIP RAISE *p. 279*
3 x 12 each side

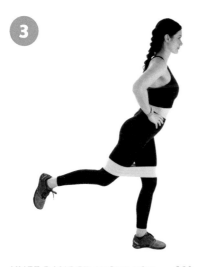

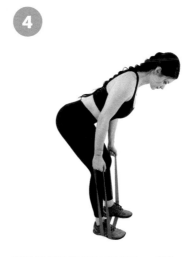

KNEE BANDED KICKBACK *p. 289*
3 x 12 each side

ROMANIAN DEADLIFT *p. 278*
4 x 15

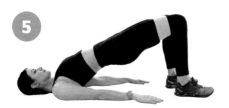

BANDED GLUTE BRIDGE *p. 285*
4 x 15

Try to perform all exercises a little slower. It is important that you feel the muscles well and perform the movement with a good execution form.

Rest between sets: 30-45 seconds.

 5 minutes COOL-DOWN

Repeat the cool-down from Monday – Lower Body 1 + Abs, Week 9, *pp. 147–148.*

SUNDAY - REST DAY

Now you can finally rest and review the past week:

- What did you learn about yourself this week?

- How were your training and nutrition?

- What is the greatest achievement you've had?

Continue to keep an eye on your nutrition and hydration.

Track the daily intake of protein, carbs, fats, vegetables, and the amount of water intake.

	Protein*	Carbs*	Fats*	Veggies*	Water*
Required portions per day					
Monday					
Tuesday					
Wednesday					
Thursday					
Friday					
Saturday					
Sunday					

*Please enter your own quantity

Next week, it's all about control and being in control of your life.

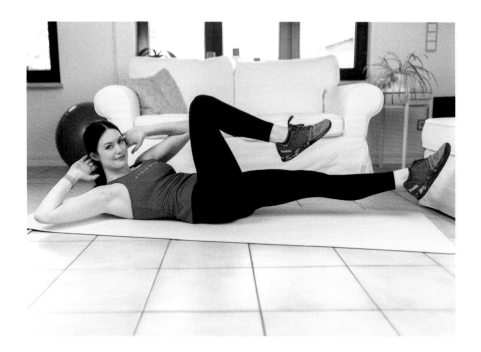

4.3.3 WEEK 11

This week, we're adding a few super sets to intensify the workouts.

> 66 *Gain control over the things you can control and learn not to get frustrated with the things you can't control.* 99

This week I have an exercise for you that will change the way you think about certain stressful situations. Maybe it will also motivate you to take action.

- Have you ever told yourself that you can't do something because you don't have time or just can't do it?

- Or have you been upset with someone because of their behavior?

If so, this exercise is for you.

Through this exercise, you will discover which things you can control and which you can't. Take a piece of paper and draw three circles.

In the smallest circle, write the things you have total control over. For example, your own actions, what you buy for dinner tonight, or what color you want the wall in your room to be.

In the middle circle, write down what you have control over to a certain degree. For example, your thoughts, your daily routine, and what time you go to bed.

And finally, in the largest circle, you write the things you have absolutely no influence on. These are the things that you cannot control. Examples: What other people think about you, how your partner behaves, what comment someone leaves on your social media, etc.

Take your time and fill in the circles with your notes. After you have filled them out, look critically at each note and ask yourself:

- Do I really have absolutely no control over it?

- Do I really have total control over it?

Spheres of control

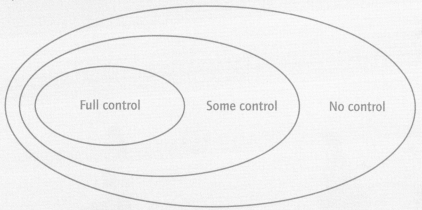

When you have done all that, look at the smallest circle. These are all the things over which you have complete control. You are the boss here. Try to keep that in mind for the next few weeks so that you can make more intentional decisions. Control what you can actually control.

Now move on to the middle circle and just think about what's there:

- What might bring these things into the smallest circle?

- What would push these things into the largest circle?

- When and how can you control these things?

- Do you even need to control these?

In the end, look at the biggest circle. These are the things you are supposed to let go of because all you can do is react to them. You can do that by using the items from the smallest circle where you have full control, such as your actions, behavior, or other factors. Learn to let go and instead focus on the things in the smallest circle.

MONDAY - LOWER BODY 1 + ABS

 WARM-UP (NO EQUIPMENT NEEDED) **5 minutes**

Repeat the warm-up from Monday - Lower Body 1 + Abs, Week 9, *pp. 143-144.*

 WORKOUT **approx. 35 minutes**

SUPERSET 1:

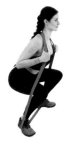

SQUAT *p. 271*
4 x 20

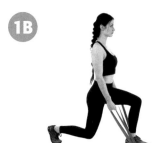

REVERSE LUNGE *p. 265*
4 x 15 each side

SUPERSET 2:

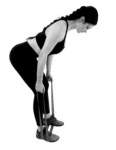

ROMANIAN DEADLIFT * *p. 278*
4 x 15

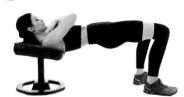

KNEE BANDED HIP THRUST * *p. 292*
4 x 20

SUPERSET 3:

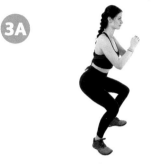

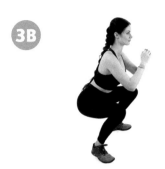

PULSE SQUAT *p. 277*
3 x 15

STATIC SQUAT HOLD *p. 280*
3 x 30-45 seconds

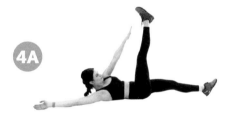

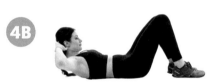

JACKKNIFE CROSSOVER *p. 259*
3 x 15 each side

CRUNCH *p. 257*
3 x AMRAP**

*   *Slowly lower the upper body in exercise 2A or the hips in exercise 2B (3-4 seconds) and quickly straighten up or lift the pelvis (1 second).*

**   *Do as many repetitions as you can. Make sure your belly stays flat and doesn't bulge or dome. If you can't hold the tension and your abdomen starts bulging, stop the exercise or take a break.*

Rest between supersets: 30-60 seconds. You should feel rested before the next superset but not completely relaxed.

 5 minutes   COOL-DOWN

Repeat the cool-down from Monday – Lower Body 1 + Abs, Week 9, *pp. 147-148.*

TUESDAY – UPPER BODY 1

 WARM-UP (NO EQUIPMENT NEEDED) **5 minutes**

Repeat the warm-up from Tuesday – Upper Body 1, Week 9 *pp. 149-150.*

 WORKOUT **approx. 25-30 minutes**

SUPERSET 1:

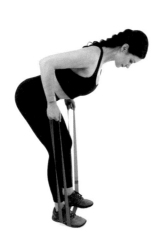   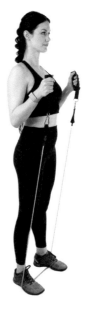

BENT-OVER ROW * *p. 254*
4 x 15

HAMMER CURL * *p. 298*
4 x 12

SUPERSET 2:

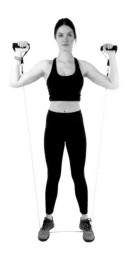

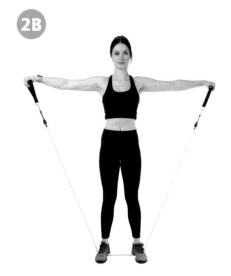

SHOULDER PRESS *p. 239*
4 x 15

LATERAL RAISE *p. 240*
4 x 12

SUPERSET 3:

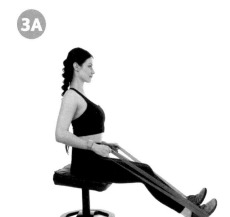

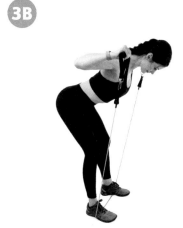

SEATED ROW * *p. 252*
3 x 15

BENT-OVER W ROW ** *p. 243*
3 x 10-15

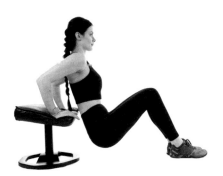

COUCH OR CHAIR DIP * *p. 300*
4 x 15

*   In the end position, when your muscles are contracted, hold the tension for 0.5-1 second before slowly lowering your arms.

**   Focus on the contracting muscles and make the movement slow and controlled. During the exercise, it is essential that you feel the back of your shoulders and that your shoulders and shoulder blades are not lifted up when pulling the band. If the band you use is too challenging, you can use a lighter weight instead, such as a water bottle or two books.

Rest between supersets: 30-60 seconds. You should feel rested before the next superset but not completely relaxed.

 COOL-DOWN   5 minutes

Repeat the cool-down from Tuesday – Upper Body 1, Week 9, *p. 153.*

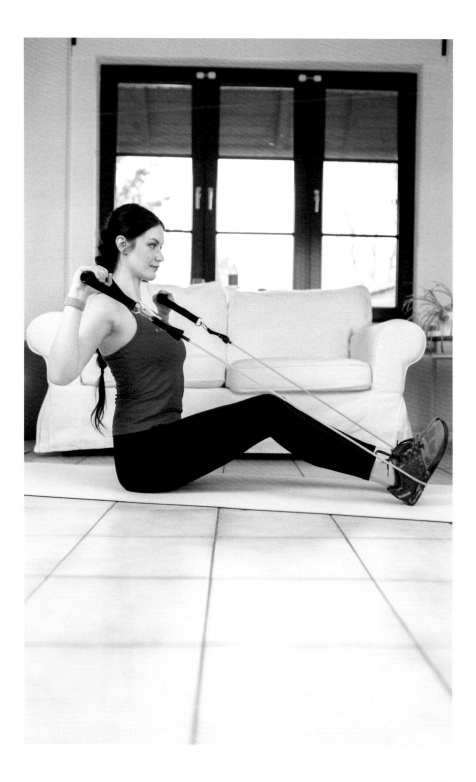

WEDNESDAY – SHOULDERS
OR ALTERNATIVELY ACTIVE REST DAY 2

If you prefer to take a break from training today, you can choose one of the following options:

- 20 minutes of light cardio exercise at a heart rate of 60%-70% of the HR_{max} (see "Tuesday – Active Rest Day" from Week 5), *p. 88.*

- "Circuit 1" from Week 5, *pp. 90-91.*

- "Circuit 2" from Week 6, *pp. 104-105.*

Alternatively, you can train your shoulders today. You can find the workout next.

 WARM-UP (NO EQUIPMENT NEEDED) **5 minutes**

Repeat this week's warm-up from Tuesday - Upper Body 1, *pp. 149-150.*

 WORKOUT **approx. 25-30 minutes**

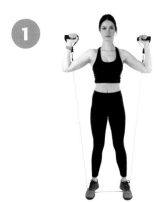

SHOULDER PRESS *p. 239*
4 x 20

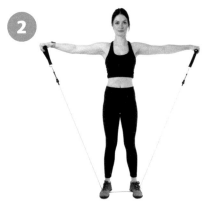

LATERAL RAISE *p. 240*
4 x 15

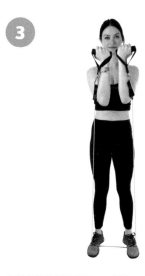

ARNOLD PRESS *p. 235*
4 x 15

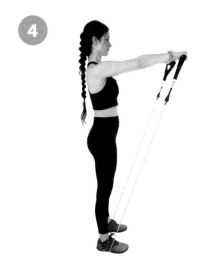

FRONT RAISE *p. 237*
4 x 12

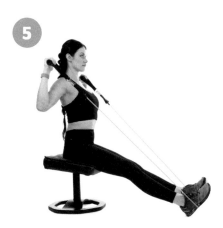

W-RUDERN IM SITZEN *p. 242*
4 x 12

Rest between sets: 30-45 seconds.

 5 minutes

COOL-DOWN

Repeat the cool-down from Wednesday – Shoulders, Week 9, *p. 156.*

THURSDAY – LOWER BODY 2 + ABS

 WARM-UP (NO EQUIPMENT NEEDED)   **5 minutes**

Repeat the warm-up from Monday – Lower Body 1 + Abs, Week 9, *pp. 143-144.*

 WORKOUT   **approx. 35 minutes**

SUPERSET 1:

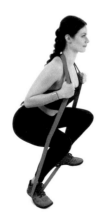

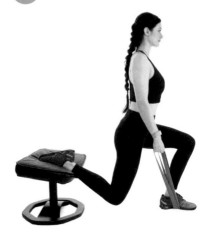

SQUAT *p. 271*
4 x 20

BULGARIAN SPLIT SQUAT *p. 266*
4 x 15 each side

SUPERSET 2:

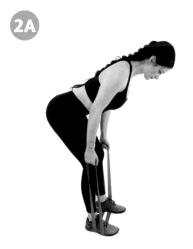

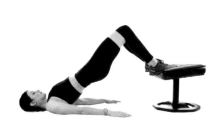

ROMANIAN DEADLIFT * *p. 278*
4 x 15

ELEVATED BANDED GLUTE BRIDGE *p. 286*
4 x 15

SUPERSET 3:

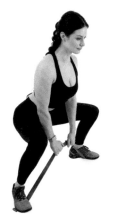

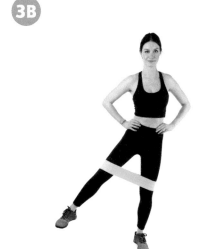

SUMO SQUAT *p. 282*
4 x 15

BANDED LEG ABDUCTION *p. 287*
4 x 15 each side

193

SUPERSET 4:

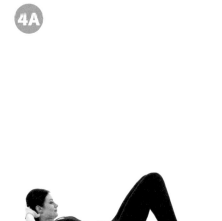

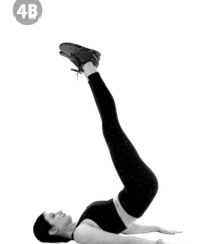

CRUNCH *p. 257*
3 x 15

REVERSE CRUNCH *p. 261*
3 x 15

* *Slow lowering of the upper body (2-3 seconds) and quick straight up (1 second).*

Rest between supersets: 30-60 seconds. You should feel rested before the next superset but not completely relaxed.

COOL-DOWN

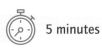 **5 minutes**

Repeat the cool-down from Monday – Lower Body 1 + Abs, Week 9, *pp. 147-148.*

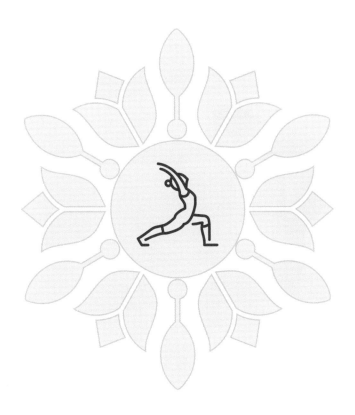

FRIDAY – UPPER BODY 2

 WARM-UP (NO EQUIPMENT NEEDED)   **5 minutes**

Repeat the warm-up from Tuesday – Upper Body 1, Week 9, *pp. 149-150.*

 WORKOUT   **approx. 25-30 minutes**

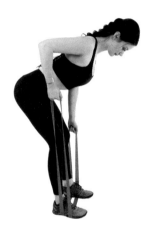

BENT-OVER SINGLE-ARM ROW *
p. 253
3 x 20 each side

SUPERSET 1:

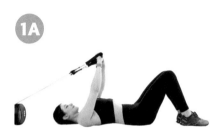

PULLOVER *p. 249*
4 x 15

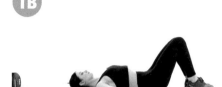

SUPINE LAT PULLDOWN *p. 251*
4 x 15

SUPERSET 2:

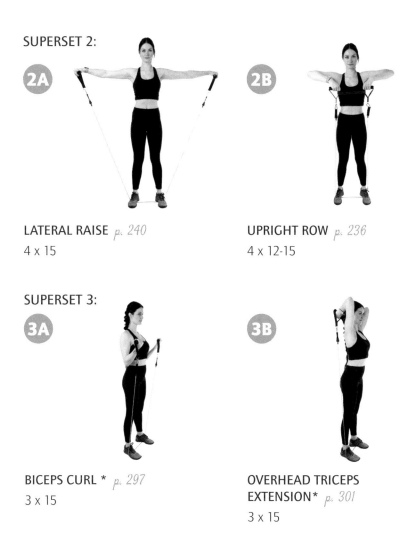

LATERAL RAISE *p. 240*
4 x 15

UPRIGHT ROW *p. 236*
4 x 12-15

SUPERSET 3:

BICEPS CURL * *p. 297*
3 x 15

**OVERHEAD TRICEPS
EXTENSION*** *p. 301*
3 x 15

*   *In the end position, when your muscles are contracted, hold the tension for
0.5 - 1 second before slowly lowering your arms.*

Rest between supersets: 30-60 seconds. You should feel rested before the next
superset but not completely relaxed.

 5 minutes   COOL-DOWN

Repeat the cool-down from Tuesday – Upper Body 1, Week 9, *p. 153.*

SATURDAY – GLUTES
OR ALTERNATIVELY ACTIVE REST DAY

If you prefer to take a break from training today, you can choose one of the following options:

- 20 minutes of light cardio exercise at a heart rate of 60-70% of the HR_{max} (see "Tuesday – Active Rest Day" from Week 5), *p. 88.*

- "Circuit 1" from Week 5, *pp. 90–91.*

- "Circuit 2" from Week 6, *pp. 104–105.*

Alternatively, you can train your glutes today. You can find the workout next.

 WARM-UP (NO EQUIPMENT NEEDED) **5 minutes**

Repeat the warm-up from Monday – Lower Body 1 + Abs, Week 9, *pp. 143–144.*

 WORKOUT **approx. 25-30 minutes**

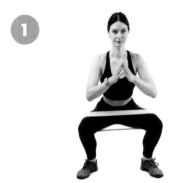

1

BANDED SQUAT WITH LEG ABDUCTION *p. 273*
4 x 20, with 10 reps each side

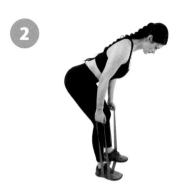

2

ROMANIAN DEADLIFT *p. 278*
4 x 15

3

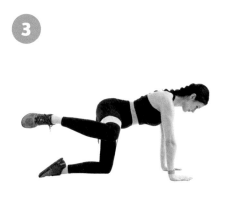

FIRE HYDRANT AND BANDED
KICKBACK *p. 293*
3 x 15 each side

4

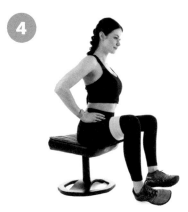

THREE-WAY SEATED BANDED
HIP ABDUCTION (STRAIGHT
UP/LEANING BACK/LEANING
FORWARD) *p. 288*
3 x 20/20/20

5

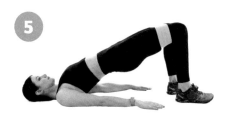

BANDED GLUTE BRIDGE * *p. 285*
3 x 15

*   *In the highest position, squeeze your glutes really hard and hold the tension for 0.5-1 second before lowering your hips.*

Try to perform all exercises a little slower. It is important that you feel the muscles well and perform the movement with a good execution form.

Rest between sets: 30-45 seconds.

 5 minutes   COOL-DOWN

Repeat the cool-down from Monday – Lower Body 1 + Abs, Week 9, *pp. 147-148.*

SUNDAY – REST DAY

Now you can finally rest and review the past week:

- What did you learn about yourself this week?

- How were your training and nutrition?

- What is the greatest achievement you've had?

Continue to keep an eye on your nutrition and hydration.

Track the daily intake of protein, carbs, fats, vegetables, and the amount of water intake.

	Protein*	Carbs*	Fats*	Veggies*	Water*
Required portions per day					
Monday					
Tuesday					
Wednesday					
Thursday					
Friday					
Saturday					
Sunday					

Please enter your own quantity

Next week, continue to try to implement all the previous recommendations consistently. Follow the philosophy of doing a little better today than yesterday. Ask yourself every day, "What can I do today a little better than yesterday?"

4.3.4 WEEK 12

Can you believe it's already the last week? One more week and you will be finished with this program. I hope you can already start to see some results. However, it's not time to relax yet. It's time to push yourself for one more week before we can analyze your results!

What can you do better this week that is within your control and that you can influence yourself?

The workout routine is the same as Week 11, but we will adjust the number of repetitions and sets.

MONDAY – LOWER BODY 1 + ABS

 WARM-UP (NO EQUIPMENT NEEDED) **5 minutes**

Repeat the warm-up from Monday – Lower Body 1 + Abs, Week 9, *pp. 143-144.*

 WORKOUT **approx. 35 minutes**

SUPERSET 1:

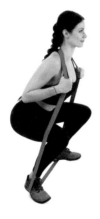

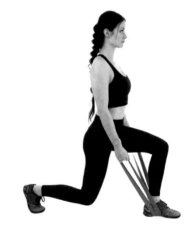

SQUAT *p. 271*
4 x 20

REVERSE LUNGE *p. 265*
4 x 15 each side

SUPERSET 2:

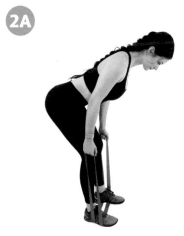

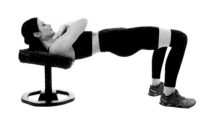

ROMANIAN DEADLIFT * *p. 278*
4 x 20

KNEE BANDED HIP THRUST * *p. 292*
4 x 20

SUPERSET 3:

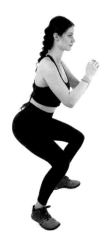

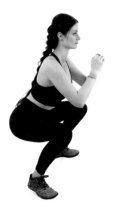

PULSE SQUAT *p. 277*
4 x 15

STATIC SQUAT HOLD *p. 280*
4 x 30-45 seconds

SUPERSET 4:

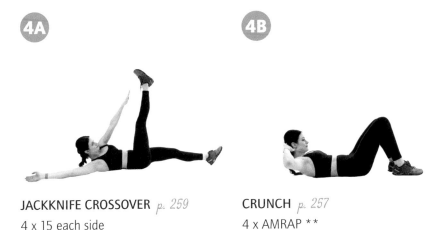

4A

4B

JACKKNIFE CROSSOVER *p. 259*
4 x 15 each side

CRUNCH *p. 257*
4 x AMRAP * *

*   *Slowly lower the upper body in exercise 2A or the hips in exercise 2B (3-4 seconds) and quickly straighten up or lift the pelvis (1 second).*

* *   *Do as many repetitions as you can. Make sure your belly stays flat and doesn't bulge or dome. If you can't hold the tension and your abdomen starts bulging, stop the exercise or take a break.*

Rest between supersets: 30-60 seconds. You should feel rested before the next supersets but not completely relaxed.

 COOL-DOWN   **5 minutes**

Repeat the cool-down from Monday – Lower Body 1 + Abs, Week 9, *pp. 147–148.*

TUESDAY – UPPER BODY 1

 5 minutes WARM-UP (NO EQUIPMENT NEEDED)

Repeat the warm-up from Tuesday – Upper Body 1, Week 9, *pp. 149-150.*

 approx. 25-30 minutes WORKOUT

SUPERSET 1:

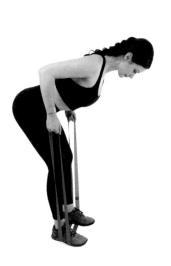

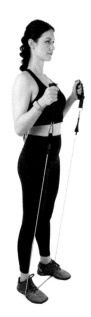

BENT-OVER ROW * *p. 254*
4 x 15

HAMMER CURL * *p. 298*
4 x 12

SUPERSET 2:

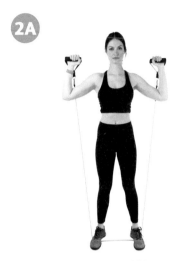

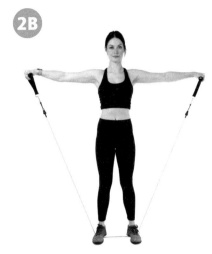

SHOULDER PRESS *p. 239*
4 x 15

LATERAL RAISE *p. 240*
4 x 12

SUPERSET 3:

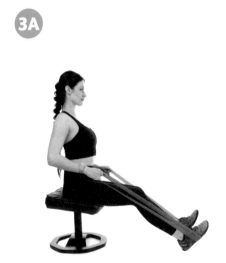

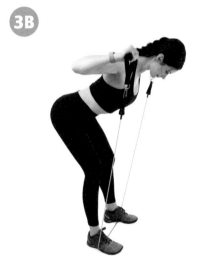

SEATED ROW * *p. 252*
4 x 15

BENT-OVER W ROW ** *p. 243*
4 x 10-15**

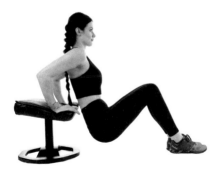

COUCH OR CHAIR DIP * *p. 300*
4 x 15

*   *In the end position, when your muscles are contracted, hold the tension for 0.5-1 second before slowly lowering your arms.*

**   *Focus on the contracting muscles and make the movement slow and controlled. During the exercise, it is essential that you feel the back of your shoulders and that your shoulders and shoulder blades are not lifted up when pulling the band. If the band you use is too challenging, you can use a lighter weight instead, such as a water bottle or two books.*

Rest between supersets: 30-60 seconds. You should feel rested before the next superset but not completely relaxed.

 5 minutes   **COOL-DOWN**

Repeat the cool-down from Tuesday – Upper Body 1, Week 9, *p. 153.*

WEDNESDAY – SHOULDERS
OR ALTERNATIVELY ACTIVE REST DAY

If you prefer to take a break from training today, you can choose one of the following options:

- 20 minutes of light cardio exercise at a heart rate of 60%-70% of the HR$_{max}$ (see "Tuesday – Active Rest Day" from Week 5), *p. 88.*

- "Circuit 1" from Week 5, *pp. 90–91.*

- "Circuit 2" from Week 6, *pp. 104–105.*

Alternatively, you can train your shoulders today. You can find the workout below.

 ## WARM-UP (NO EQUIPMENT NEEDED) **5 minutes**

Repeat this week's warm-up from Tuesday – Upper Body 1, *pp. 149–150.*

 ## WORKOUT **approx. 25-30 minutes**

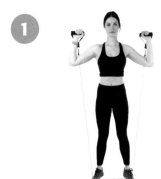

SHOULDER PRESS *p. 239*
4 x 20

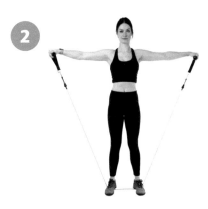

LATERAL RAISE *p. 240*
4 x 15

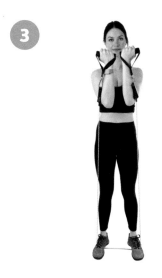

ARNOLD PRESS p. 235
4 x 15

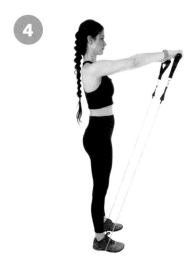

FRONT RAISE p. 237
4 x 12

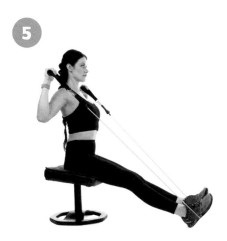

SEATED W ROW p. 242
4 x 12

Rest between sets: 30-45 seconds.

 5 minutes　　　　　　　　　　　　**COOL-DOWN**

Repeat the cool-down from Wednesday – Shoulders, Week 9, p. 156.

THURSDAY – LOWER BODY 2 + ABS

 WARM-UP (NO EQUIPMENT NEEDED)   **5 minutes**

Repeat the warm-up from Monday – Lower Body 1 + Abs, Week 9, *pp. 143-144.*

 WORKOUT   **approx. 35 minutes**

SUPERSET 1:

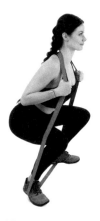

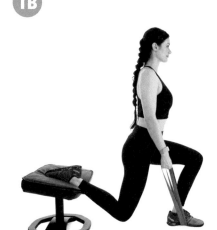

SQUAT *p. 271*
4 x 20

BULGARIAN SPLIT SQUAT *p. 266*
4 x 15 each side

SUPERSET 2:

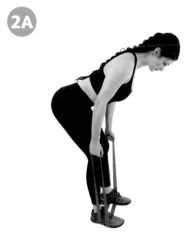

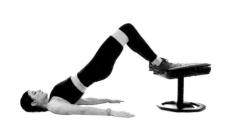

ROMANIAN DEADLIFT * *p. 278*
4 x 20

ELEVATED BANDED GLUTE BRIDGE *p. 286*
4 x 15

SUPERSET 3:

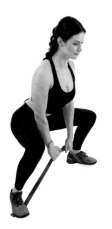

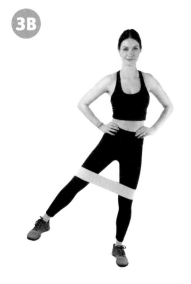

SUMO SQUAT *p. 282*
4 x 20

BANDED LEG ABDUCTION *p. 287*
4 x 15 each side

SUPERSET 4:

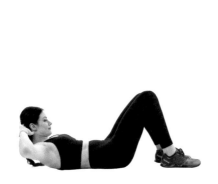

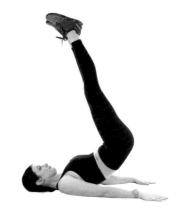

CRUNCH *p. 257*
4 x 15

REVERSE CRUNCH *p. 261*
4 x 15

*   *Slow lowering of the upper body (2-3 seconds) and quick straight up (1 second).*

Rest between supersets: 30-60 seconds. You should feel rested before the next superset but not completely relaxed.

COOL-DOWN

  5 minutes

Repeat the cool-down from Monday – Lower Body 1 + Abs, Week 9, *pp. 147–148.*

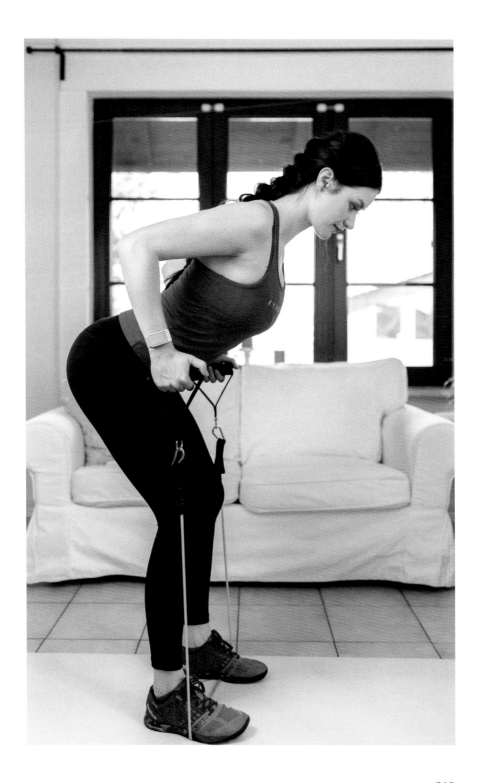

FRIDAY – UPPER BODY 2

 WARM-UP (NO EQUIPMENT NEEDED) **5 minutes**

Repeat the warm-up from Tuesday – Upper Body 1, Week 9, *p. 149–150.*

 WORKOUT **approx. 25-30 minutes**

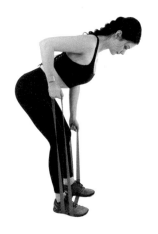

**BENT-OVER SINGLE-ARM
ROW *** *p. 253*
4 x 20 each side

SUPERSET 1:

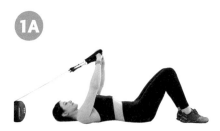

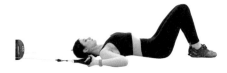

PULLOVER *p. 249*
4 x 20

SUPINE LAT PULLDOWN *p. 251*
4 x 15

SUPERSET 2:

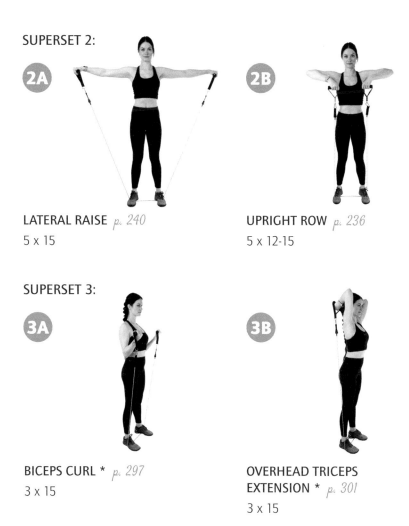

LATERAL RAISE *p. 240*
5 x 15

UPRIGHT ROW *p. 236*
5 x 12-15

SUPERSET 3:

BICEPS CURL * *p. 297*
3 x 15

**OVERHEAD TRICEPS
EXTENSION *** *p. 301*
3 x 15

* *In the end position, when your muscles are contracted, hold the tension for
0.5-1 second before slowly lowering your arms.*

Rest between supersets: 30-60 seconds. You should feel rested before the next
superset but not completely relaxed.

 5 minutes

COOL-DOWN

Repeat the cool-down from Tuesday – Upper Body 1, Week 9, *p. 153.*

215

SATURDAY – GLUTES
OR ALTERNATIVELY ACTIVE REST DAY

If you prefer to take a break from training today, you can choose one of the following options:

* 20 minutes of light cardio exercise at a heart rate of 60%-70% of the HR_{max} (see "Tuesday – Active Rest Day" from Week 5), *p. 88.*

* "Circuit 1" from Week 5, *pp. 90–91.*

* "Circuit 2" from Week 6, *pp. 104–105.*

Alternatively, you can train your glutes today. You can find the workout next.

 WARM-UP (NO EQUIPMENT NEEDED)   **5 minutes**

Repeat the warm-up from Monday – Lower Body 1 + Abs, Week 9, *pp. 143–144.*

 WORKOUT   **approx. 30-35 minutes**

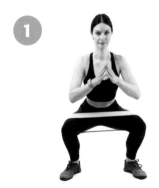

BANDED SQUAT WITH LEG ABDUCTION *p. 273*
4 x 20, with 10 reps each side

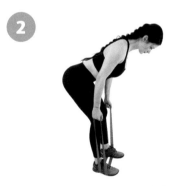

ROMANIAN DEADLIFT *p. 278*
4 x 20

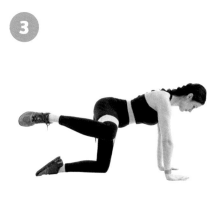

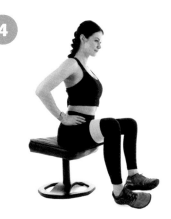

FIRE HYDRANT AND BANDED KICKBACK *p. 293*

4 x 15 each side

THREE-WAY SEATED BANDED HIP ABDUCTION (STRAIGHT UP/LEANING BACK/LEANING FORWARD) *p. 288*

3 x 30/30/30

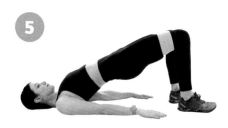

BANDED GLUTE BRIDGE * *p. 285*

4 x 15

* *In the highest position, squeeze your glutes really hard and hold the tension for 0.5-1 second before lowering your hips.*

Try to perform all exercises a little slower. It is important that you feel the muscles well and perform the movement with a good execution form.

Rest between sets: 30-45 seconds.

 5 minutes COOL-DOWN

Repeat the cool-down from Monday – Lower Body 1 + Abs, Week 9, *p. 147-148.*

SUNDAY - REST DAY

You made it through, congratulations! You can be very proud of yourself, and I hope you enjoyed this program. Hopefully, you have also been monitoring your nutrition this week.

Track the daily intake of protein, carbs, fats, vegetables, and the amount of water intake.

	Protein*	Carbs*	Fats*	Veggies*	Water*
Required portions per day					
Monday					
Tuesday					
Wednesday					
Thursday					
Friday					
Saturday					
Sunday					

Please enter your own quantity

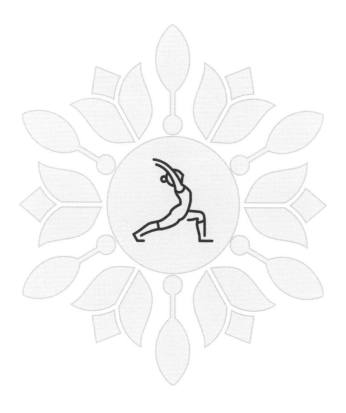

5

PROGRESS ASSESSMENT

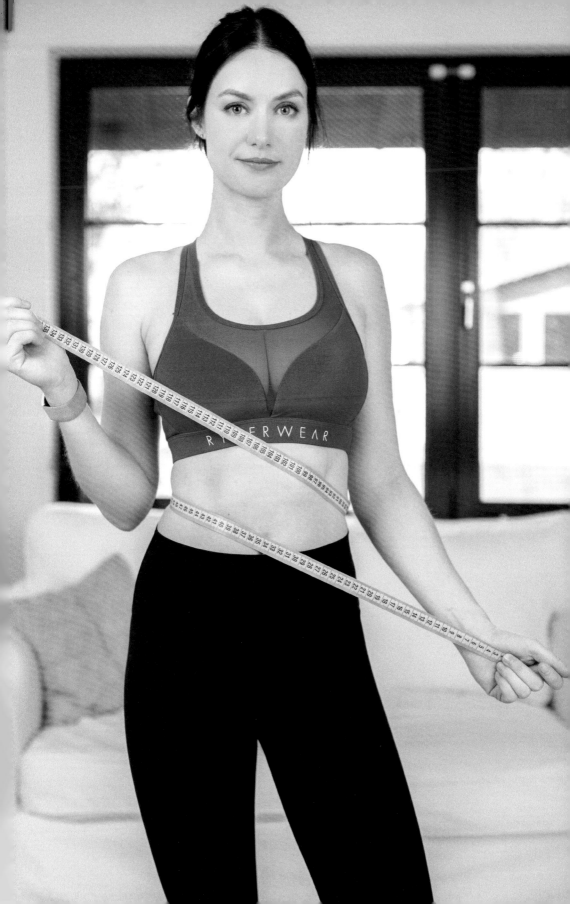

5 PROGRESS ASSESSMENT

Now you can capture your progress and analyze your results.

- What have you learned about yourself over the past 12 weeks?
- What has changed for you?
- What do you do better now?
- What could you do even better?

Just like at the beginning of the program, weigh yourself in the morning right after you get up and after you go to the bathroom. Please do not drink or eat anything before that.

Once you have weighed yourself, please take the comparison photos. Again, it is best to take one photo from the side, one with your back, and one with your face in front of the camera. To compare the pictures better, try wearing the same clothes as you did in the first photos. Also, try to make sure that the lighting is similar.

In addition, you can also take different body measurements if you took them at the beginning of the program: chest, waist, hips, and the circumference of your arms and legs.

From the photos, you can easily see the differences in your body.

- Does your skin look different?
- Do your clothes fit a little looser?

Pay attention to your body silhouette and your posture.

 NOTE

Feel free to share your results with me! Send me a quick message via email, tag @mamafitnesscoaching or @elenabiedert in your photos on Instagram, or share it in our Facebook community. Let's connect and cheer each other all the way!

5.1 How do you interpret the results and the changes regarding your weight and body measurements?

Has your weight not changed but your body circumferences are smaller?

This means you now have less fat mass and more muscle mass. In other words, you have improved your body composition. By the way, this is also why you should never interpret weight alone and should not focus too much on the scale reading.

Did your weight go up? Your body measurements also went up a notch, but in the photos, you have a better shape (rounder shoulders and glutes, for example), or do your clothes fit better?

This means that you most likely gained muscle mass.

Has your weight dropped and body circumferences reduced?

This means that you have lost weight or fat mass.

At the end of the day, all that matters is that you're happy with the results. However, if they are not what you had hoped for, ask yourself the following questions:

1. "Did I really do everything as instructed in the program?"

2. "Did I adjust my diet according to the recommendations?"

3. "Was I absolutely consistent with my diet, and did I track all snacks, sauces, dressings, and oils?"

If you answered "yes" to these three fundamental questions but your results aren't as good as you'd expected – they're there, but not as significant – just give your body time. Twelve weeks is a reasonable amount of time to lay the initial foundation for the physique you want and to incorporate new habits into your daily routine. Nonetheless, that's still a very short period of time to make drastic changes.

Be patient, and always remember that all the small improvements will become huge if you stay consistent. You will get much closer to your goals if you stay even 50%-70% perfect and 100% consistent for an extended period (Precision Nutrition Inc.).

An example of this: You are not too strict in your diet. You understand and follow the basics of a balanced diet and allow yourself treats as well. Your workout is also not perfect. Sometimes you don't even get to it because the day was so stressful. A few days later, however, you pick up where you left off. You find a balance between load, stress, and recovery. Training and nutrition are no longer a must for you but rather part of your everyday life.

If you are 100% perfect only 50% of the time, however, it will not get you far.

An example of this: If you train for one month and stick very strictly to your nutrition plan, but then don't train again for a month and eat all kinds of things. Or even if you keep putting your training on pause and returning to old eating habits when you get a little stressed or feel like you don't have time. The usual mindset here is: "Next Monday, next month, or as soon as life gets back to 'normal,' I'll continue."

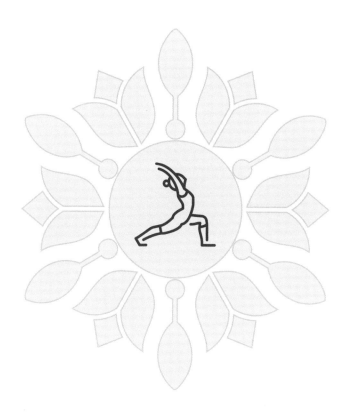

6

OUTLOOK

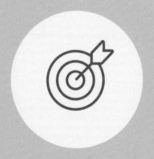

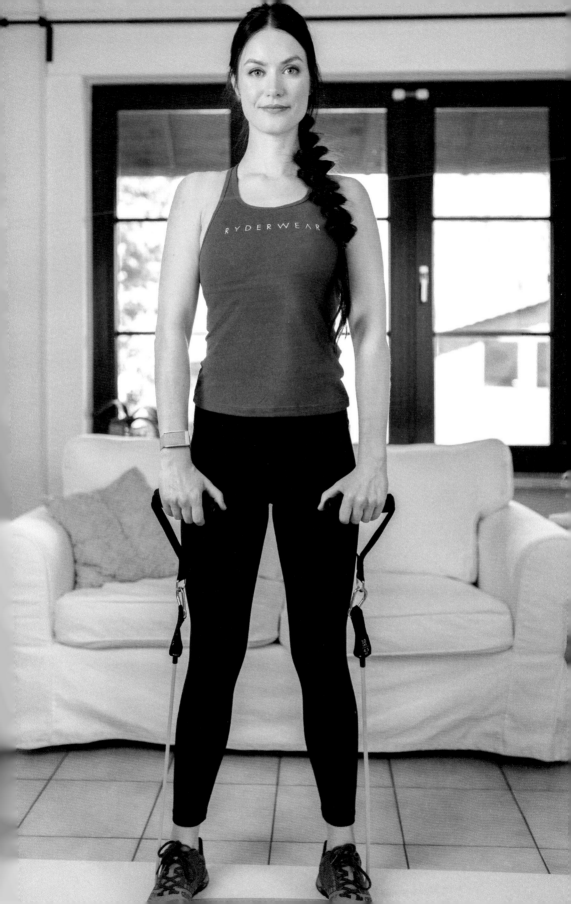

6 OUTLOOK

You've completed your training program and are wondering *what now*?

Here's what you can do next:

- You could start the program over. Since you've gotten stronger over the 12 weeks, you just need to adjust the resistance used at the beginning of the program.

- You could also start another program and continue with the dietary changes. However, no matter what program you follow next, I suggest you take a few days to recover and either do no training at all or only light workouts. This will help your body to recover and regenerate, not only physically but also mentally.

- If you're looking for a new program and a more personalized approach to your training and nutrition program with regular check-ins and adjustments, I also offer one-on-one virtual coaching. You can find out more on my website: **mamafitnesscoaching.com**. Additionally, I offer programs and coaching for expecting and new moms.

- As far as your nutrition and goals are concerned, I recommend not jumping from one goal to the next too quickly. For example, don't switch between weight loss and muscle gain every few weeks. Jumping back and forth will only decrease your progress. Stay consistent over a longer period of time and be patient because big changes take time.

- Finally, if you have any questions or need more support, feel free to contact me by email at elena@mamafitnesscoaching.com or through my social networks. My Instagram accounts are @elenabiedert and @mamafitnesscoaching.

Free Coaching and Gifts

Are you interested in learning about nutrition, fitness, and motherhood? Well, I've got some exciting news for you! Each month, I share free, bite-sized educational videos on these topics, and to sweeten the deal, I'm also giving away a free gift related to the topic discussed in the video. Don't miss out on this fantastic opportunity to learn and receive free goodies! Follow the URL: **mamafitnesscoaching.com/5-minutes-coaching-with-elena**

Don't miss out on all the exciting updates, challenges, and gifts! Stay in the loop by subscribing to my newsletter right now: **eepurl.com/gOhnSz**

Community

Ready to join a supportive community of like-minded people and get all your questions about fitness and nutrition answered quickly? Our private Facebook group is the place to be! Whether you're a new parent or just looking to improve your health, you'll get exclusive access to tips, challenges, and resources to help you reach your goals. Join us now!

www.facebook.com/groups/mamafitnesscoaching

Supplements

Are you after top-notch supplements that can help you reach your fitness goals? Look no further than Kaged! Every batch is third-party tested for quality and free of artificial flavors and colors. Order now at **kaged.com** and get 15% off by using code Elena15 at checkout.

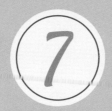

GLOSSARY

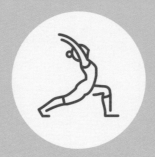

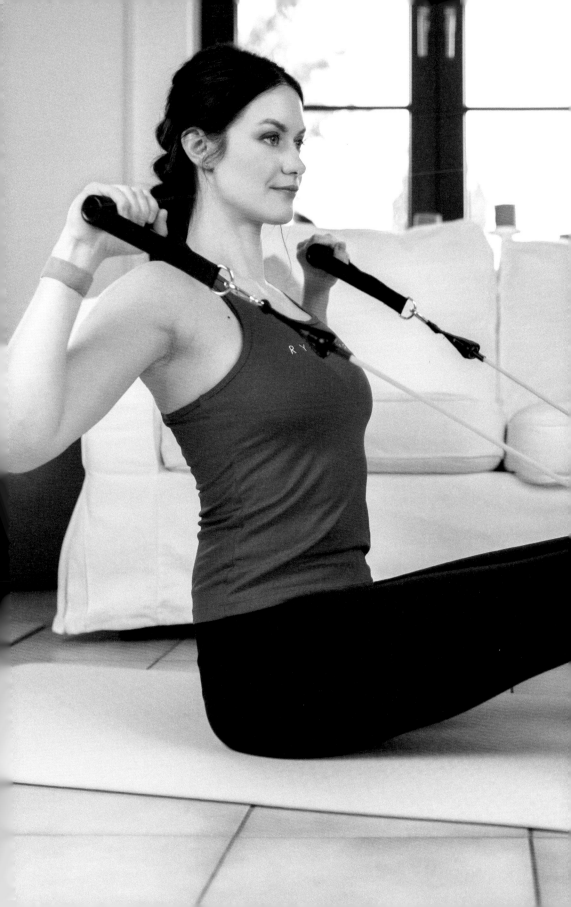

7 GLOSSARY

In the glossary, you will find definitions of the terminology used in the book and descriptions of the correct execution for all exercises from the training program presented in chapter 4. This way, you can quickly look them up at any time.

Terms are sorted alphabetically. The exercise catalog is sorted according to the muscle groups being trained.

You can also watch a video for each exercise. All you have to do is scan the QR code with your smartphone. With modern smartphones, you simply open your camera app and point it at the code. Alternatively, if you have an older smartphone, you can download a QR scanner app and use it to access the videos.

7.1 Terminology and definitions

Mindful eating is neither a new diet nor a form of nutrition. Mindfulness has its roots in Buddhism and can be applied to all forms of life. It is about how we deal with ourselves and the world. This includes our attitude toward and exploration of our diet and eating habits.

Active rest means that you don't do any strength training that day, but try to stay active as much as possible. For example, you could jog, ride a bike, walk, or swim for 20 minutes. Alternatively, you can do a workout that is not as intense as your other workouts but will still provide some exercise.

AMRAP – as many reps as possible.

The eccentric phase is when you give in to the resistance in a controlled manner, for example, when you lower your hips during the squats.

The concentric phase is when you push against the resistance, such as standing up from a squat.

Macronutrients include proteins, carbohydrates, and fats. These are the nutrients from which the body obtains energy.

Micronutrients, on the other hand, are substances such as vitamins and minerals that have no energy value but are essential for the body to function.

Neutral spine - in the neutral position, the spine has its natural double-S curve, which serves to absorb impact.

Progressive Overload refers to the progressive increase in your power output. This refers to the rise in the workload that you expose your body to.

Rest day means you can just put your feet up and relax. You're not supposed to do any workouts on that day.

"Black-and-white thinking" - foods are often divided into good and bad categories. However, there are no good or bad foods. They only differ in their macro- or micronutrients.

A superset consists of two exercises performed one after the other without rest. Suppose a superset consists of exercises A and B, each with three sets and 15 repetitions. In that case, this means that you first perform a set of 15 repetitions of exercise A and then a set of 15 repetitions of exercise B without resting in between. That would be one set in your superset. After finishing one superset, you can take the rest as stated in your workout. After the rest, you start the second set of the superset and so on until you have finished all supersets.

Circuit - in a circuit, all exercises are performed one after the other within the specified time without a break. After a short break, you can repeat the circuit if it is scheduled in the training program.

7.2   List of exercises

SHOULDERS

Alternating Front and Lateral Raise

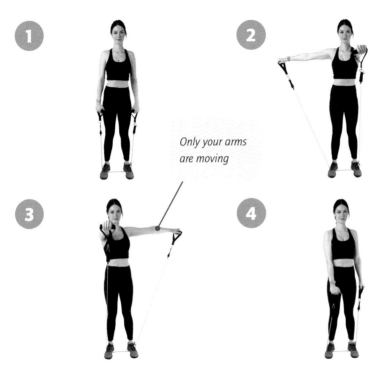

Only your arms are moving

- Stand up straight holding the band handles.

- While exhaling, raise your arms straight.

- While inhaling, shift the arms by 90 degrees in front of you.

- Lower the arms on the next exhale. This is one repetition.

- Repeat the same in the other direction.

Here you can see the video demo.

Arnold Press

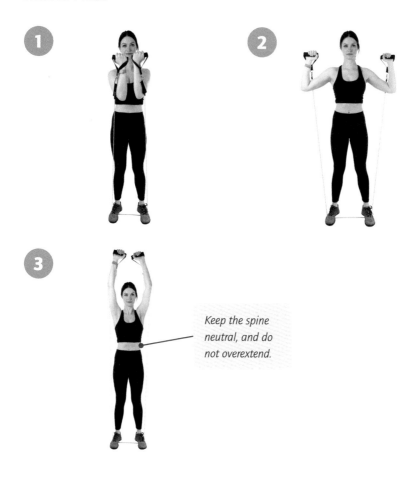

Keep the spine neutral, and do not overextend.

- Stand straight with the band handles at chest level and palms facing your body.

- Extend your arms as you exhale while turning your wrists over. In the end position, your palms face away from you.

- As you inhale, return to the starting position. At the same time, turn your wrists toward you again.

Here you can see the video demo.

235

Upright Row

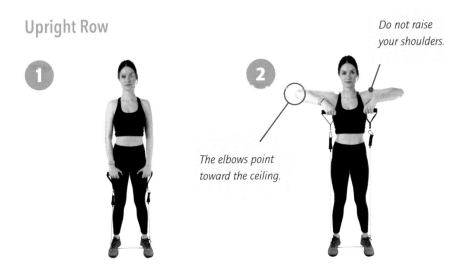

Do not raise your shoulders.

The elbows point toward the ceiling.

- Stand up straight with the band handles in your hands. The palms of your hands touch your thighs.

- As you exhale, pull the band straight up until your hands are about level with your chin. Keep the band close to your body while your elbows point toward the ceiling or parallel to the floor.

- As you inhale, slowly lower the band back to the starting position.

Here you can see the video demo.

Front Raise

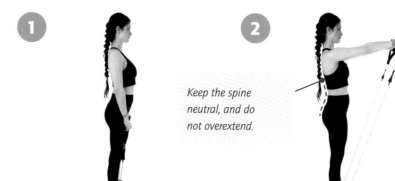

Keep the spine neutral, and do not overextend.

- Stand up straight with the band handles in your hands.

- As you exhale, raise your stretched arms up in front of you.

- Lower your arms as you inhale.

Here you can see the video demo.

Behind-the-Neck Press

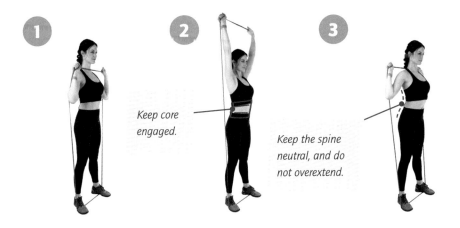

Keep core engaged.

Keep the spine neutral, and do not overextend.

- Stand up straight with the band in your hands.

- Bring the band handles over your shoulders so your elbows are bent and your forearms are perpendicular to the floor.

- As you exhale, push your arms straight up. Do not lift your shoulders.

- As you inhale, slowly lower your arms so the band is behind your neck.

- On the next repetition, bring the band forward again, alternating with each repetition.

- If you lack flexibility, you can do the "Shoulder Press" exercise instead.

Here you can see the video demo.

Shoulder Press

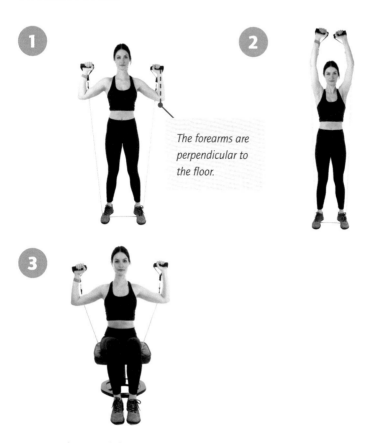

The forearms are perpendicular to the floor.

- Stand up straight with the band handles in your hands.

- Bring the band handles over your shoulders so your elbows are bent and your forearms are perpendicular to the floor.

- As you exhale, push your arms straight up. Do not lift your shoulders.

- As you inhale, slowly lower your arms back to the starting position. You can also do the exercise while sitting (see position 3).

Here you can see the video demo.

Lateral Raise

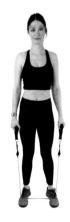

Keep your neck relaxed.

The wrists are in line with the elbows or slightly lower.

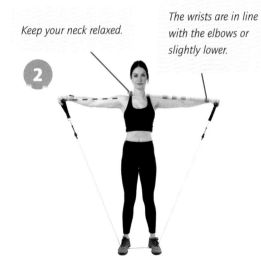

- Stand up straight with the band handles in your hands.

- As you exhale, raise your straight arms up to the sides.

- Lower your arms as you inhale.

Here you can see the video demo.

Bent-Over Lateral Raise

Pull with your rear delts.

Keep the spine neutral, and do not overextend.

- Bend forward and hold the band handles in your hands. Keep your spine neutral.

- Exhaling, raise your extended arms up over the sides.

- Lower your arms as you inhale.

- Engage your rear delts as you do this.

Here you can see the video demo.

Seated W Row

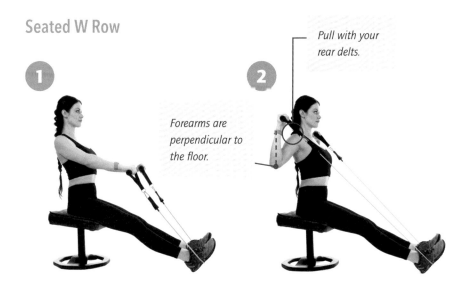

Pull with your rear delts.

Forearms are perpendicular to the floor.

- Sit on a chair or floor and hold the band handles in your hands.

- As you exhale, pull the band over your sides toward your head until your arms form a "W" shape with your head.

- As you inhale, slowly return to the starting position.

- While doing this, make sure you engage the back of your shoulders and your upper back.

Here you can see the video demo.

Bent-Over W Row

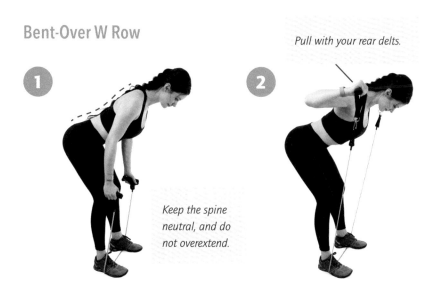

Pull with your rear delts.

Keep the spine neutral, and do not overextend.

- Bend forward and hold the band handles in your hands.

- As you exhale, pull the band over your sides toward your head until your arms form a "W" shape with your head.

- As you inhale, slowly return to the starting position.

- While doing this, make sure you engage the back of your shoulders and your upper back.

Here you can see the video demo.

Seated Y Raise

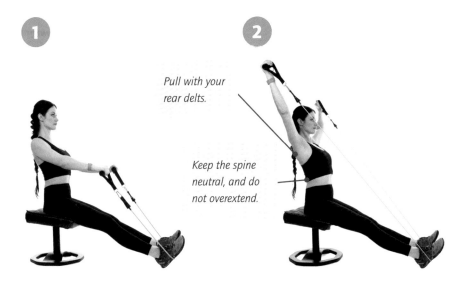

Pull with your
rear delts.

Keep the spine
neutral, and do
not overextend.

- Sit on the chair or bench and hold the band handles in your hands.

- As you exhale, raise your arms diagonally up to your sides until your arms form a "Y" shape with your upper body.

- As you inhale, slowly return to the starting position.

- While doing this, make sure you engage the back of your shoulders and your upper back.

Here you can see the video demo.

CHEST

Seated Chest Press

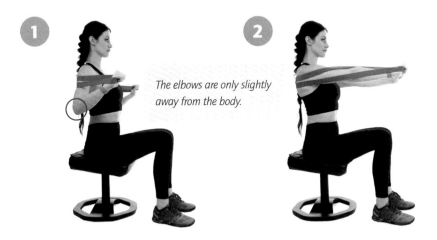

The elbows are only slightly away from the body.

- Sit on a chair or on the floor, place the center of the band behind your back at chest level and hold the ends. Your hands should be at chest level with your elbows slightly away from the sides of your body.

- As you exhale, press the handles or ends of the band forward and together at the same time.

- As you inhale, slowly bring your arms back to the starting position.

Here you can see the video demo.

Narrow Push-Up

See "Triceps".

Fly

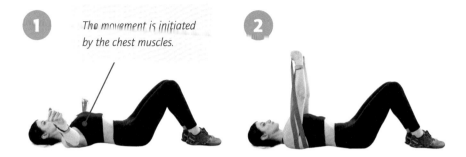

- Lie on the floor. Place the center of the band under your back at chest level and hold the ends. Arms are slightly bent at the elbows and are perpendicular to the sides of the torso.

- As you exhale, bring your arms together in front of you. The chest muscles initiate the movement, and the arms remain slightly bent at the elbows.

- As you inhale, slowly lower your arms back down over your sides. Always keep a slight tension in your chest and arms until you have completed all repetitions.

Here you can see the video demo.

Seated Fly

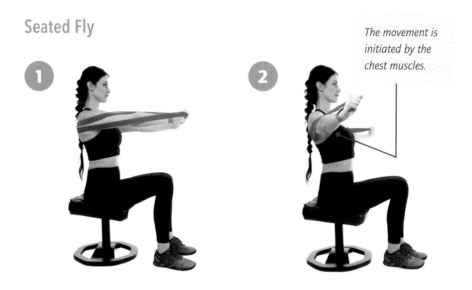

The movement is initiated by the chest muscles.

- Sit on a chair or on the floor. Place the center of the band behind your back at chest level and hold the ends. Your arms are slightly bent at the elbows and are extended in front of you at chest level and perpendicular to your torso.

- As you inhale, slowly bring your arms apart to your sides until they are almost perpendicular to your torso.

- As you exhale, slowly bring your arms back together in front of you. The chest muscles initiate the movement, and your arms remain slightly bent at the elbows. Always keep a slight tension in your chest and arms until you have completed all repetitions.

Here you can see the video demo.

Push-Up

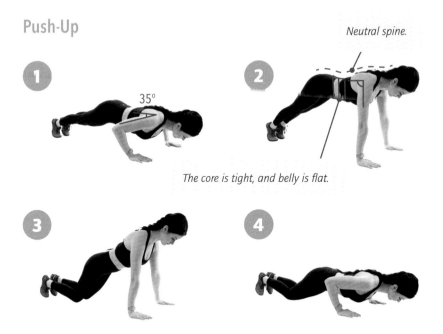

Neutral spine.

35°

The core is tight, and belly is flat.

- In the prone position, stretch out your body. Place your hands on the floor about shoulder-width apart at chest height. Your fingers point forward, and your upper arms are at a 35-degree angle from your body.

- As you exhale, straighten your arms, pressing your body up. Make sure you squeeze your chest muscles while you perform this movement.

- Weight is evenly distributed on your toes and hands. Your head, neck, spine, glutes, and knees form a line, and your core is tight.

- As you inhale, bend your elbows and bring your body back down until you are just inches from the floor.

- If the exercise is too difficult, you can also do it on your knees (see 3 and 4). Alternatively, you can place your upper body higher, for example, on the couch or even against the wall.

Here you can see the video demo.

Pullover

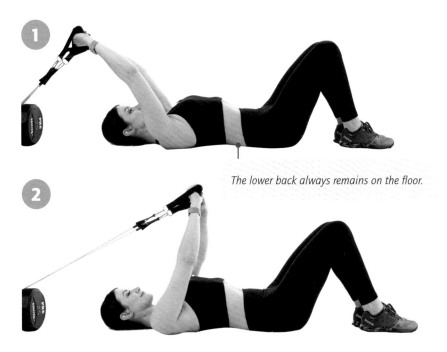

The lower back always remains on the floor.

- Make sure your resistance band is well secured. Lie on the floor and take the handles in your hands. The band should be slightly loose.

- As you exhale, pull your arms over your head toward your legs up to chest level. Your arms should be extended but slightly bent at the elbows, Both the chest and back muscles will be actively working during the movement.

- Slowly bring the straightened arms back up behind the head as you inhale. If you can attach the band somewhere at the top, for example, on a door, you can also do this exercise while standing.

Here you can see the video demo.

BACK

Single-Arm Row

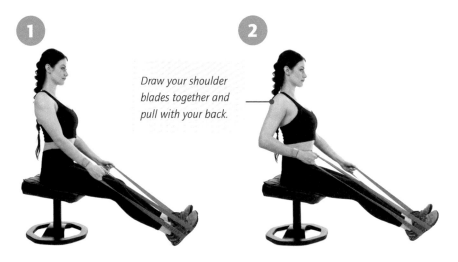

Draw your shoulder blades together and pull with your back.

- Sit on the floor with your legs extended or slightly bent at the knees. Hold the band in your hands, with the center of the band around your feet. Make sure you keep your spine in its neutral position and your core engaged.

- As you exhale, pull the band toward you with one arm until your hand is close to your body. Start the movement by drawing your shoulder blades back. Make sure you pull the band with your back muscles not your arm.

- As you inhale, slowly extend your arm back to the starting position.

Here you can see the video demo.

Supine Lat Pulldown

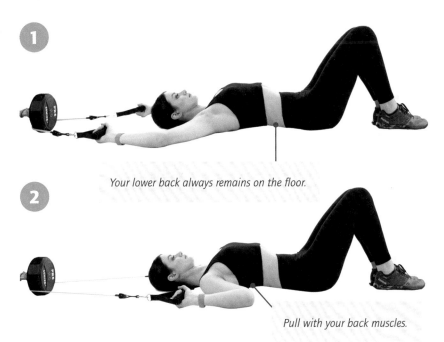

Your lower back always remains on the floor.

Pull with your back muscles.

- Make sure your fitness band is well secured. Lie on the floor and take the band in your hands. The band should be slightly loose.

- As you exhale, draw your shoulder blades together and pull your arms down to your sides. Your arms should glide along the floor. The whole movement is initiated by your back muscles.

- As you inhale, slowly bring your arms back up. If you can attach the band somewhere at the top, such as on a door, you can also do this exercise while standing.

Here you can see the video demo.

Seated Row

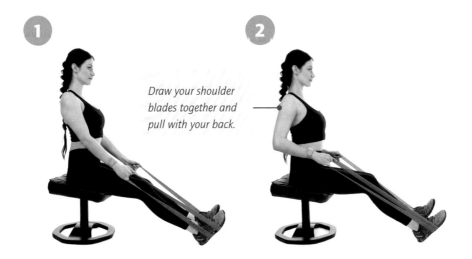

Draw your shoulder blades together and pull with your back.

- Sit on the floor with your legs extended or slightly bent at the knees. Hold the band in your hands, with the center of the band around your feet. Make sure you keep your spine in its neutral position and your core engaged.

- As you exhale, pull the band toward you until your hands are close to your body. Start the movement by drawing your shoulder blades back. Make sure you pull the band with your back muscles, not your arms.

- As you inhale, slowly extend your arms back to the starting position.

Here you can see the video demo.

Good Morning

See "Glutes".

Sumo Deadlift

See "Legs".

Bent-Over Single-Arm Row

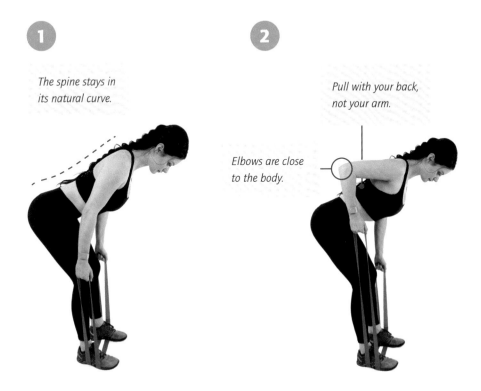

- Take the band in your hands and bend forward. Keep your back straight so that your spine remains in its natural curve.

- As you exhale, pull the end of the band toward your chest with one arm. As you do so, draw your shoulder blades back and bend your arm at the elbow. Make sure you pull the band with your back muscles, not your arm.

- Hold the position briefly, then slowly extend your arm again as you inhale.

- In one set, do all the repetitions for one arm first, then for the other arm.

Here you can see the video demo.

Bent-Over Row

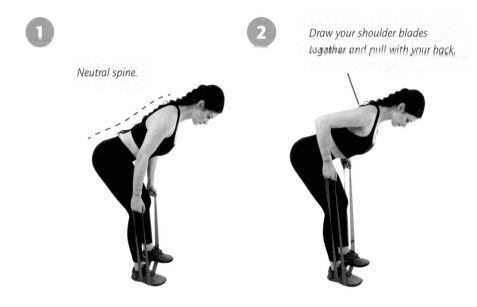

• Take the band in your hands and bend forward. Keep your back straight so that your spine remains in its natural curve.

• As you exhale, pull the ends of the band toward your chest. As you do so, draw your shoulder blades together and bend your arms at the elbow. Make sure you pull the band with your back muscles, not your arms.

• Hold the position briefly, then slowly extend your arms again as you inhale.

Here you can see the video demo.

Bent-Over Row With Supinated Grip

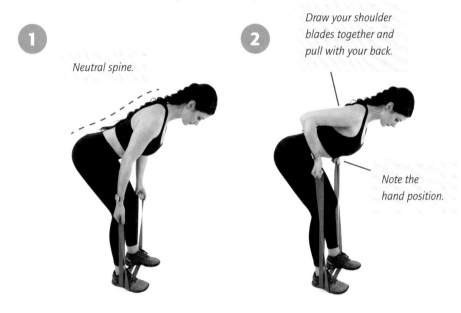

Neutral spine.

Draw your shoulder blades together and pull with your back.

Note the hand position.

- Take the band in your hands with the palms facing away from your body and bend forward. Keep your back straight so that your spine remains in its natural curve.

- As you exhale, pull the ends of the band toward your chest. As you do so, draw your shoulder blades together and bend your arms at the elbow. Make sure you pull the band with your back muscles, not your arms.

- Hold the position briefly, then slowly extend your arms again as you inhale.

Here you can see the video demo.

Pullover

See "Chest".

Seated W Row

See "Shoulders".

Bent-Over W Row

See "Shoulders".

Seated Y Raise

See "Shoulders".

ABS

Crunch

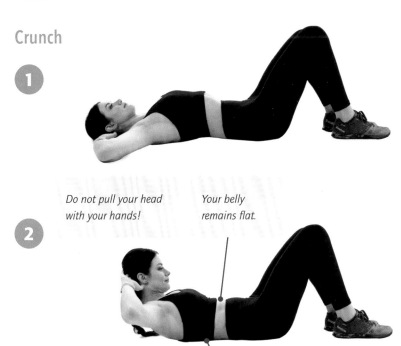

Do not pull your head with your hands!

Your belly remains flat.

Your middle and lower back remain on the floor.

- Lie with your back on the floor. You can keep your hands under your head, but be careful not to pull your head forward with your hands during the exercise!

- Roll your chest up off the mat as you exhale. As you do this, the distance between the top of your pelvis and the bottom of your rib cage will be shortened. Make sure your belly always stays flat and doesn't bulge outward.

- As you inhale, slowly lower your chest to the floor, but don't lose the abdominal tension completely.

Here you can see the video demo.

Standing Opposite Elbow-to-Knee Crunch

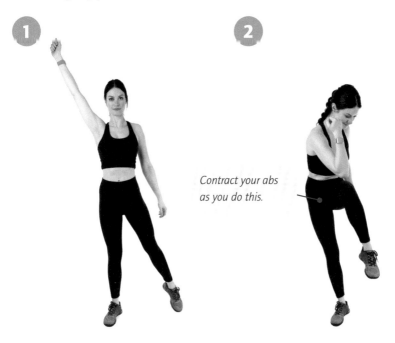

Contract your abs as you do this.

- Stand upright with your legs shoulder-width apart so that your right arm is up in the air and your left arm is relaxed at the side of your body. Alternatively, you can place your hands loosely on the back of your head.

- On the exhale, lift the left knee explosively while rotating the upper body to the left until you touch or almost touch the bent knee with the right elbow.

- As you inhale, return to the starting position, and repeat the same movement for the other side.

- You can alternate sides or do all the repetitions for one side and then all the repetitions for the other side.

Here you can see the video demo.

Jackknife Crossover

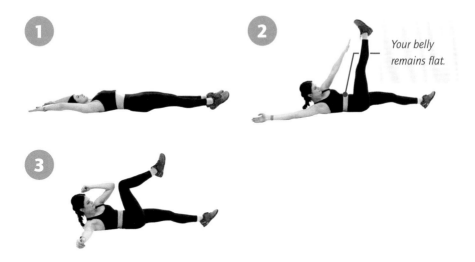

Your belly remains flat.

- Lie on your back on the floor with your legs and arms extended.

- As you exhale, bring your straight leg and straight arm together diagonally.

- As you inhale, slowly bring the arm and leg back to the starting position. Keep your abs under tension while doing this. Make sure that your belly always stays flat and does not bulge outward. If this happens, perform the exercise with bent legs and arms (see position 3).

- You can alternate sides or do all the repetitions for one side and then all the repetitions for the other side.

Here you can see the video demo.

Standing Elbow-to-Knee Crunch

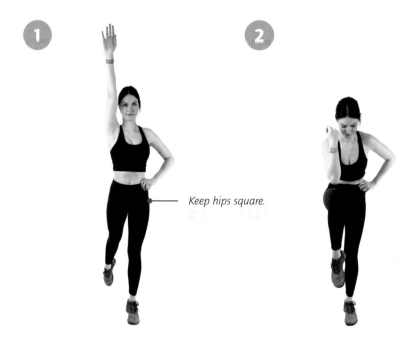

Keep hips square.

- Stand upright with your legs shoulder-width apart. Straighten the right arm up, the left hand resting on the hip. As you inhale, bring your right leg back and raise it slightly into the air, keeping your left leg slightly bent.

- As you exhale, bring your right knee and elbow together explosively in front of your belly while rounding your back.

- As you inhale, straighten up again.

- Do all the repetitions for one side first and then for the other.

Here you can see the video demo.

Reverse Crunch

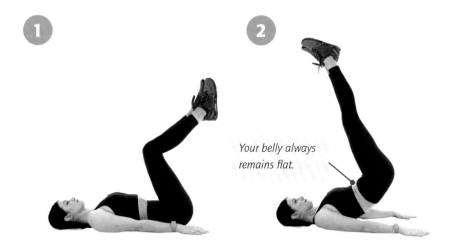

Your belly always remains flat.

- Lie with your back on the floor and bend your knees to form a square angle.

- Now lift your hips off the floor as you exhale and stretch your legs toward the ceiling.

- Hold this position briefly and slowly lower your hips back down on the inhale.

Here you can see the video demo.

Side Plank

Your belly always remains tight and flat.

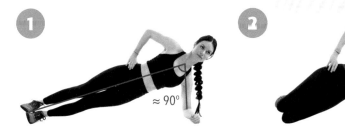

- Lie on the floor on your side, supporting your upper body on your forearm. Engage your core and, as you exhale, lift your pelvis until your body forms a straight line from head to toe.

- Hold this position for as long as stated in the program. Keep the tension steady and breathe normally into the chest.

- If the position is too difficult with extended legs, you can lean on your knees instead (see position 2).

Here you can see the video demo.

Elbow Plank

The belly always remains tight and flat.

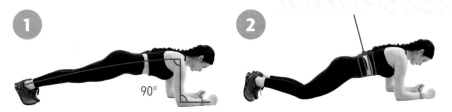

- Get into a prone position on the floor, supporting your weight on your toes and forearms. The body should form a straight line from the shoulders to the feet, your core muscles should be tight, and your belly should always remain flat and not bulge outwards.

- Hold this position for as long as stated in the program. Keep the tension steady and breathe normally into the chest only.

- If the position is too difficult with extended legs, you can lean on your knees instead (see position 2).

Here you can see the video demo.

Mountain Climber

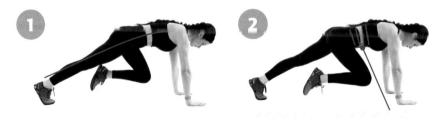

Your belly always remains tight and flat.

- Take the push-up position with your hands just below your shoulders. Your whole body should be in a straight line with a tight core.

- Jump off the floor with your right foot and bring your right knee to your chest. Then straighten the leg again and jump off with the left foot.

- Perform these explosive jumps, alternating between legs, keeping your whole body straight and your belly flat. Breathe normally into the chest.

Here you can see the video demo.

LEGS

Reverse Lunge

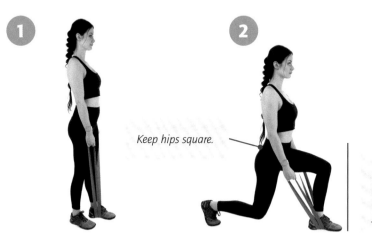

Keep hips square.

Your knee doesn't go beyond your toes.

- Stand upright with your legs shoulder-width apart and hold the band in your hands.

- As you inhale, bring one leg back. Your knee should remain above your ankle and not go beyond your toes.

- As you exhale, bring the leg back to the starting position. Keep your core tight, and make sure your pelvis doesn't tilt to the side.

- Repeat for the other leg. You can alternate legs or do all repetitions for one leg and then for the other.

Here you can see the video demo.

Banded Leg Abduction

See "Glutes".

Bulgarian Split Squat

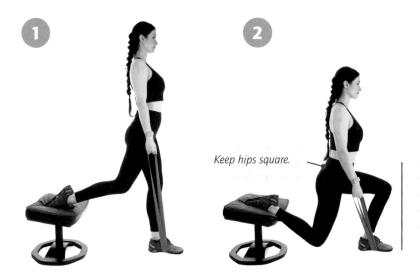

Keep hips square.

The knee doesn't go beyond the toes.

- Stand upright with your legs shoulder-width apart and hold the band in your hands. Then place one leg on the elevation behind you, for example, on a chair.

- As you inhale, bend your front leg at the knee. While doing this, the knee of the front leg should stay above your ankle and not go beyond your toes. Lower the knee of the back leg.

- As you exhale, straighten your front leg again. Keep your core tight, and make sure your pelvis doesn't tilt sideways.

Here you can see the video demo.

Single-Leg Deadlift

 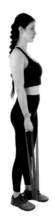

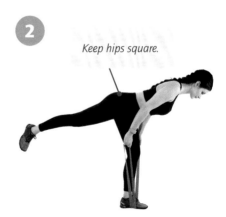

Keep hips square.

- Stand upright with your legs shoulder-width apart and hold the band in your hands.

- As you inhale, lower your upper body forward while lifting one leg behind you. Your upper body and raised leg should be parallel or almost parallel to the floor. Make sure your pelvis doesn't tilt sideways or rotate. The leg on the floor is slightly bent at the knee.

- As you exhale, bring your back leg to the floor and straighten your torso. Maintain body tension and initiate the entire movement from the hips.

- Make sure that your spine remains in its natural position.

Here you can see the video demo.

Jump Squat

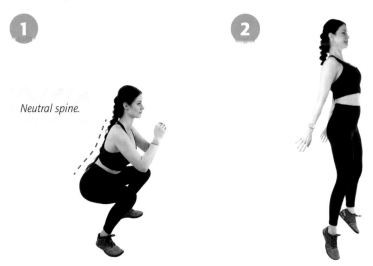

Neutral spine.

- Stand upright with your legs shoulder-width apart.

- As you inhale, slowly bend your knees and lower your hips until your thighs are parallel to the floor. Make sure your knees do not collapse inward and your spine remains in its natural position.

- As you exhale, explosively push your body back up over the center of your foot, lifting your feet off the ground.

Here you can see the video demo.

Jumping Jack

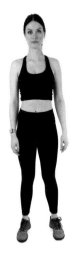

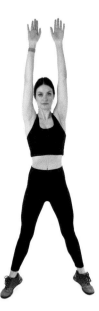

- Stand up straight. Your hands hang to the sides of your body.

- Then explosively lift your extended arms up over your head and simultaneously jump into a wide stance with your legs.

- Then jump back to the starting position. This is one repetition.

- Breathe normally while doing this.

Here you can see the video demo.

High Knee Bounce Skip

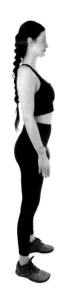
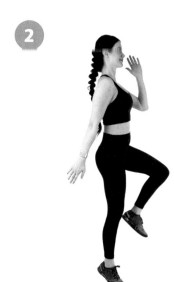

- Stand upright with your legs shoulder-width apart. Explosively pull your right knee up until the thigh is roughly parallel to the floor. At the same time, pull your left arm, which is bent at a square angle, up until the upper arm is roughly parallel to the floor. Your left leg remains extended, and your foot leaves the ground briefly.

- After landing on your right foot, repeat the same movement with your left leg. Alternate sides repeatedly.

Here you can see the video demo.

Squat

 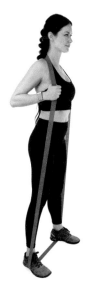

Neutral spine.

 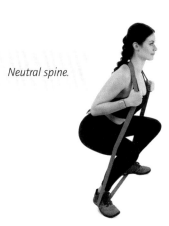

- Stand upright with your legs shoulder-width apart and hold the band. The band should be at the same height on both sides.

- As you inhale, slowly bend your knees, and lower your hips until your thighs are parallel to the floor. Make sure your knees do not collapse inward and your spine remains in its natural position.

- As you exhale, push your body back up over the center of your foot.

Here you can see the video demo.

Chair or Box Squat

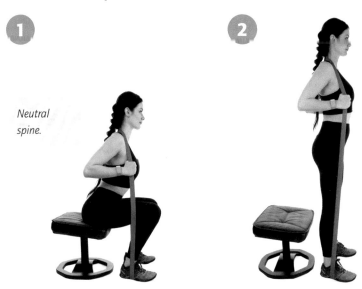

Neutral spine.

- Stand upright with your legs shoulder-width apart in front of a chair and hold the band.

- As you inhale, slowly bend your knees, and lower your hips until they touch the chair. You can sit down on the chair, but make sure that you do not lose body tension and the spine remains in its natural position.

- As you exhale, push your body back up over the center of your foot.

Here you can see the video demo.

Banded Squat With Leg Abduction

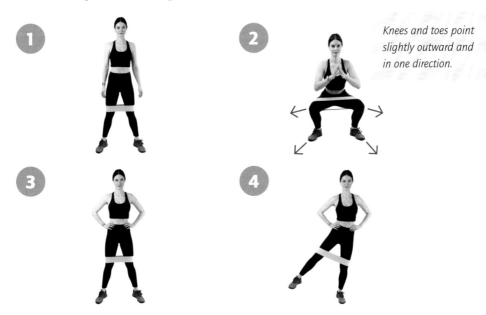

Knees and toes point slightly outward and in one direction.

- Place the band directly over your knees and stand upright with your legs shoulder-width apart.

- As you inhale, slowly bend your knees, and lower your hips until your thighs are parallel to the floor. Make sure your knees do not collapse inward and that your spine remains in its natural position throughout the exercise.

- As you exhale, quickly push your body back up over the center of your foot until you are completely upright. Then immediately lift one leg up to the side. This part of the movement is initiated by the muscles of the side of the leg and your glutes.

- Repeat with the other leg. You can alternate legs repeatedly or do all repetitions with one leg first and then all repetitions with the other leg.

Here you can see the video demo.

Front Squat

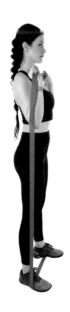

Neutral spine.

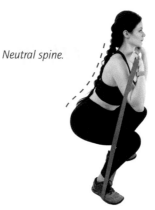

- Stand upright with your legs shoulder-width apart and hold the band in front of your chest. The band should be at the same height on both sides.

- As you inhale, slowly bend your knees, and lower your hips until your thighs are parallel to the floor. Make sure your knees do not collapse inward and your spine remains in its natural position.

- As you exhale, push your body back up over the center of your foot.

Here you can see the video demo.

Curtsy Lunge

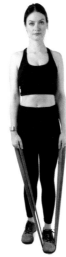

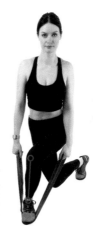

Keep hips square.

Your knee is above your ankle.

- Stand upright with your legs shoulder-width apart and hold the band in your hands.

- As you inhale, bring one leg diagonally back. As you do so, your front knee should remain right above your ankle and not pass the toes.

- As you exhale, bring your leg back to the starting position. Make sure your core is tight, and your pelvis doesn't tilt sideways.

- Repeat with the other leg. You can alternate legs or do all repetitions for one leg and then for the other.

Here you can see the video demo.

High Knees

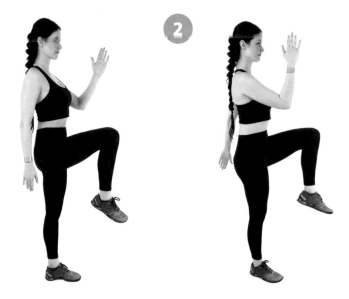

- Stand upright with legs shoulder-width apart. Explosively pull your right knee up to chest height. Then step onto your toes with your left foot. Both arms swing along as if marching.

- Your right leg returns to the floor, and you repeat with the other leg. Alternate legs quickly and explosively as if running fast on the spot.

Here you can see the video demo.

Pulse Squat

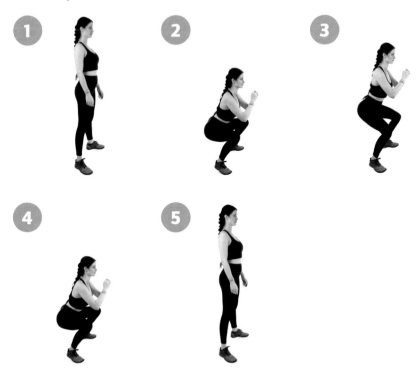

- Stand upright with your legs shoulder-width apart.

- As you inhale, slowly bend your knees, and lower your hips until your thighs are parallel to the floor. Make sure your knees do not collapse inward and your spine remains in its natural position.

- When deep in the squat, raise your hips just a few inches and lower them back into the squat again.

- After that, you stand up again on the exhale by pushing your body over the center of the foot.

Note: You can also do this exercise with a band.

Here you can see the video demo.

Romanian Deadlift

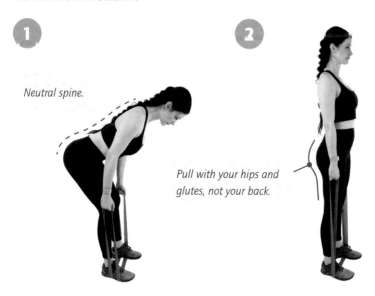

Neutral spine.

Pull with your hips and glutes, not your back.

- As you inhale, slowly lower your upper body until your hands are just below your knees. Always keep your spine in a neutral position.

- As you exhale, bring your torso back up by pushing your hips forward and extending your knees. Keep the band close to your body throughout the movement. The movement is initiated from the hips and glutes.

Here you can see the video demo.

Side-Lying Hip Raise

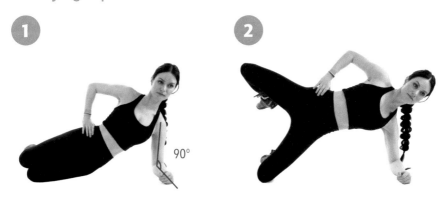

- Lie on the floor on your side, supporting your upper body on your forearm. Your legs are bent at the knees.

- Tighten your core and lift your pelvis as you exhale, supporting yourself on your knee and raising your other bent leg. Try to bring your legs as far apart as possible.

- As you inhale, lower your hips back to the floor.

Here you can see the video demo.

279

Static Squat Hold

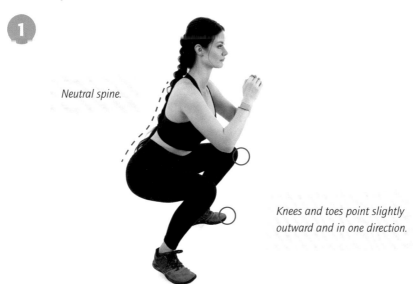

Neutral spine.

Knees and toes point slightly outward and in one direction.

- Get into a squat position while maintaining your core tension. Your thighs are roughly parallel to the floor.

- Now hold this position for the given time.

Here you can see the video demo.

Step-up

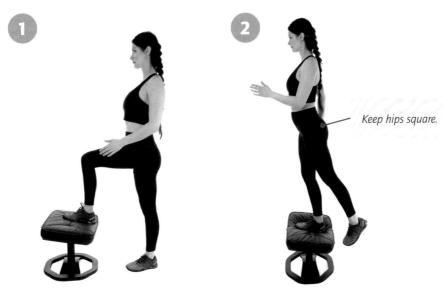

Keep hips square.

- Stand upright with your legs shoulder-width apart.

- As you inhale, place one foot on the step in front of you (e.g., on a stair or on a chair), and as you exhale, step up onto the chair. As you do this, the knee of your forward leg should stay right above your ankle and not go beyond your toes. Make sure your core holds the tension and your pelvis does not tilt sideways.

- As you inhale, slowly return to the starting position.

- Repeat with the other leg. You can alternate legs repeatedly or do all repetitions for one leg first and then all repetitions for the other leg.

- The higher the object you step on, the more difficult the exercise will be. You can also perform the exercise with a band.

Here you can see the video demo.

Sumo Squat

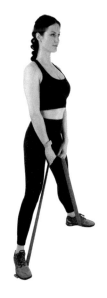

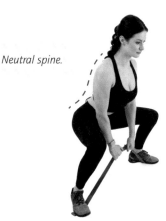

Neutral spine.

- Stand upright with your legs at double shoulder width. Your toes point slightly outward. Hold the band in your hands.

- As you inhale, slowly bend your knees, and lower your hips until your thighs are parallel to the floor. Make sure your knees do not collapse inward and your spine remains in its natural position.

- As you exhale, push your body back up over the center of your foot. The movement is initiated from your legs and glutes.

Here you can see the video demo.

Sumo Deadlift

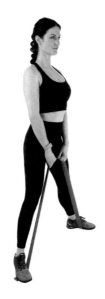

Neutral spine.
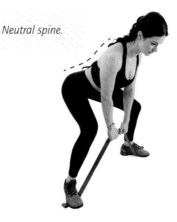

- Stand upright with your legs at double shoulder width. The toes point slightly outward. Hold the band in your hands.

- As you inhale, slowly lower your upper body. At the same time, bend your knees slightly. Make sure that your spine remains in its natural position.

- As you exhale, push your hips forward and straighten your upper body and legs. The movement is initiated from your hips.

Here you can see the video demo.

GLUTES

B-Stance Glute Bridge

The belly remains flat.

1

2

Squeeze your glutes hard.

- Lie on your back and position your feet so that one foot is entirely on the floor. This leg carries almost the entire body weight. The other foot moves slightly forward and only touches the floor with the heel. The heel is roughly in line with the toe of the weight-bearing foot.

- As you exhale, push your hips up, squeezing your glutes as hard as possible in the highest position. Make sure your belly stays flat and does not bulge outward.

- As you inhale, lower your hips back down.

- Repeat with the other leg. First, do all repetitions for one leg and then do all repetitions for the other leg.

Here you can see the video demo.

Banded Glute Bridge

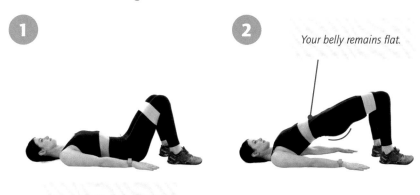

Your belly remains flat.

Squeeze your glutes hard.

- Lie on your back and place the band directly over your knees.

- As you exhale, push your hips up, squeezing your glutes as hard as possible in the highest position. Make sure your belly stays flat and does not bulge outward. Your feet should be placed so that your knees are directly above your ankles.

- As you inhale, lower your hips back down.

Here you can see the video demo.

Elevated Banded Glute Bridge

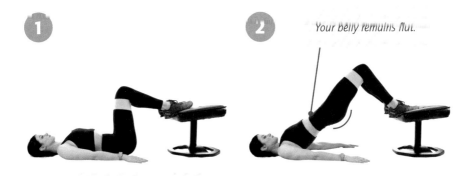

Your belly remains flat.

Squeeze your glutes hard.

- Lie on your back and place the band directly over your knees. Place your feet on an elevation, such as stairs or a chair.

- As you exhale, push your hips up, squeezing your glutes as hard as possible in the highest position. Make sure your belly stays flat and does not bulge outward.

- As you inhale, lower your hips back down.

Here you can see the video demo.

Banded Leg Abduction

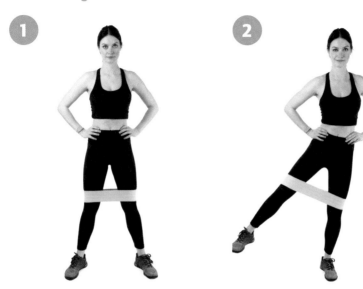

- Stand upright and place the band directly over your knees. Place your hands on your hips or hold on to an object for stability.

- As you exhale, lift one leg sideways at a slight angle backward. The movement is mainly initiated from the glutes.

- As you inhale, slowly lower your leg back down.

- Repeat with the other leg. First, do all repetitions for one leg and then for the other.

Here you can see the video demo.

Three-Way Seated Banded Hip Abduction (Straight Up/Leaning Back/Leaning Forward)

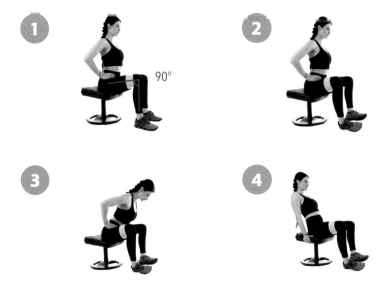

- Place the band directly over your knees and sit on a chair or stool so your legs are bent at a square angle. Your upper body is straight.

- Now bring your legs apart by pressing your knees against the band. You can also roll your feet outward for greater amplitude. The movement is initiated from the hips or glutes. Then bring your knees back to the starting position and perform the given number of repetitions. You should perform the exercise in a controlled manner, but you can also do it very quickly.

- Now lean back and repeat the given number of repetitions.

- Now lean forward and repeat the given number of repetitions.

Here you can see the video demo.

Knee Banded Kickback

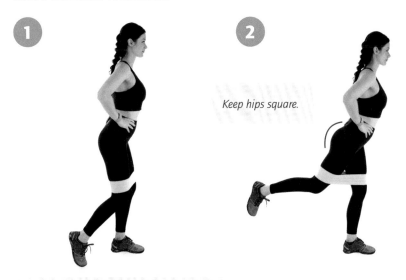

Keep hips square.

The movement is initiated from the glutes.

- Stand upright and place the band directly over your knees. Place your hands on your hips or hold on to an object for stability.

- As you exhale, lift one leg backward. The movement is mainly initiated from the glutes.

- On the inhale, slowly lower the leg back down.

- Repeat with the other leg. First, do all repetitions for one leg and then for the other.

Here you can see the video demo.

Bulgarian Split Squat

See "Legs".

Single-Leg Deadlift

See "Legs".

Hip Thrusts

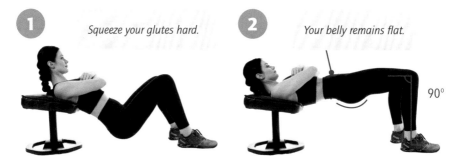

Squeeze your glutes hard.

Your belly remains flat.

90°

- Lie with your back on an elevation (e.g., on a couch).

- As you exhale, push your hips up, squeezing your glutes as hard as possible in the highest position. Make sure your belly stays flat and does not bulge outward. Your feet should be placed so your knees are directly above your ankle and your shins at a square angle with your thighs. Your back should be placed on the elevation so that the bottom edge of your shoulder blades is on the edge of the elevation, like on the edge of the couch.

- As you inhale, lower your hips back down.

Here you can see the video demo.

B-Stance Hip Thrust

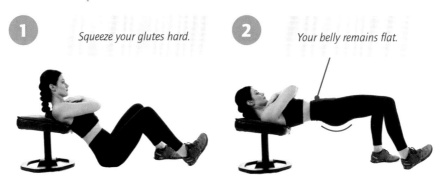

① *Squeeze your glutes hard.*   ② *Your belly remains flat.*

- Lie with your back on an elevation (e.g., on a couch) and position your feet so that one foot is entirely on the floor. This leg carries almost the entire body weight. The other foot is slightly forward and only touching the floor with the heel. The heel is roughly in line with the toe of the weight-bearing foot.

- As you exhale, push your hips up, squeezing your glutes as hard as possible in the highest position. Make sure your belly stays flat and does not bulge outward. Your feet should be placed so that your knees are directly above the ankle and your shins at a square angle with your thighs. Your back should be placed on the elevation so that the bottom edge of your shoulder blades is on the edge of the elevation, like on the edge of the couch.

- As you inhale, lower your hips back down.

Here you can see the video demo.

Knee Banded Hip Thrust

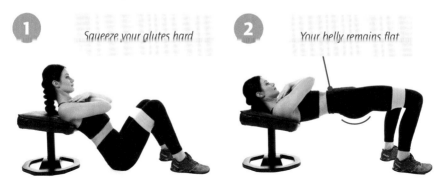

- Just like "Hip Thrusts", but place the band directly over your knees.

Here you can see the video demo.

Banded Squat With Leg Abduction

See "Legs".

Fire Hydrant and Banded Kickback

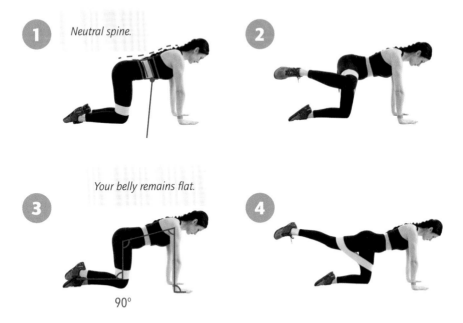

- Position the band directly above your knees and take a quadruped stance. Your thighs and arms are perpendicular to the floor. Your core is tight.

- As you exhale, lift your leg up to the side. The leg is still bent at the knee at 90 degrees. Make sure your upper body does not rotate and remains parallel to the floor.

- As you inhale, lower your leg to the floor.

- As you exhale, lift your leg backward. The leg is still bent at a 90-degree angle at the knee. Make sure you do not overextend your lower back.

- As you inhale, lower your leg to the floor.

- This is one repetition. Repeat with the other leg. You can alternate the legs or do all repetitions for one leg first and then for the other.

Here you can see the video demo.

Frog Pump

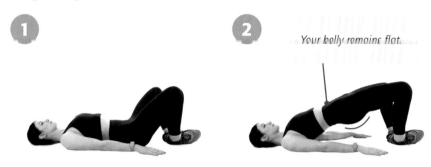

Your belly remains flat.

- Lie on your back and place your feet so that the soles of your feet touch each other. The feet are about the same distance from the body as in the "Glute Bridge" or "Hip Thrust" exercises.

- As you exhale, push your hips up, squeezing your glutes as hard as possible in the highest position. Make sure your belly stays flat and doesn't bulge outward.

- As you inhale, lower your hips back down.

Here you can see the video demo.

Pulse Squat

See "Legs".

Romanian Deadlift

See "Legs".

Good Morning

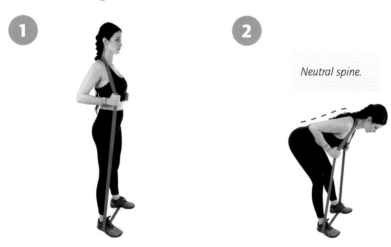

Neutral spine.

- Stand upright on the band and place the band on your neck as low as possible.

- As you inhale, bring your hips back and, at the same time, lower your upper body down as far as you can. Your spine should remain in its natural curve, with your knees slightly bent.

- As you exhale, push your hips forward powerfully and straighten out your whole body again.

Here you can see the video demo.

Side-Lying Hip Raise

See "Legs".

Step-up

See "Legs".

Sumo Squat

See "Legs".

Sumo Deadlift

See "Legs".

BICEPS

Biceps Curl

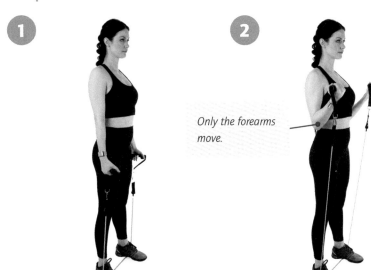

Only the forearms move.

- Stand upright and hold the band. Your palms face each other.

- As you exhale, bend your arms and simultaneously rotate your wrists so that your palms are pointed in the direction of your face in the final position. Your upper arms and elbows do not move. Only your forearms move.

- As you inhale, lower your arms back down.

Here you can see the video demo.

Hammer Curl

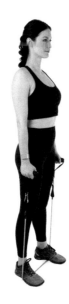

Only the forearms move.

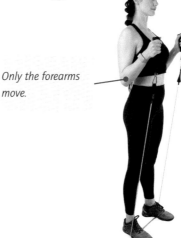

- Stand upright and hold the band. Your palms face each other throughout the entire movement.

- As you exhale, bend your arms. Your upper arms and elbows do not move. Only your forearms move.

- As you inhale, lower your arms back down.

Here you can see the video demo.

Biceps Curl With Pronated Grip

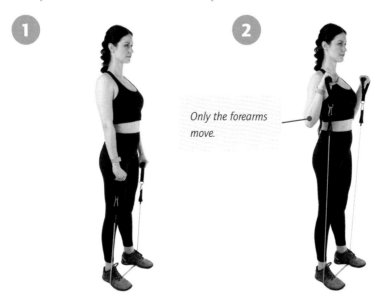

Only the forearms move.

- Stand upright and hold the band. Your palms point backward.

- As you exhale, bend your arms. Your upper arms and elbows do not move. Only your forearms move.

- As you inhale, lower your arms back down.

Here you can see the video demo.

TRICEPS

Couch or Chair Dip

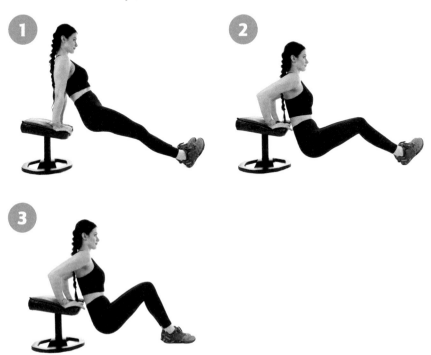

- Place your palms on the couch or chair with your fingers facing your body. Position your feet in front of you so that your thighs are parallel to the floor.

- As you inhale, bend your arms at the elbows and simultaneously lower your hips until your upper arms are roughly parallel to the floor.

- As you exhale, push your entire body weight up through your arms and straighten your arms.

Here you can see the video demo.

Overhead Triceps Extension

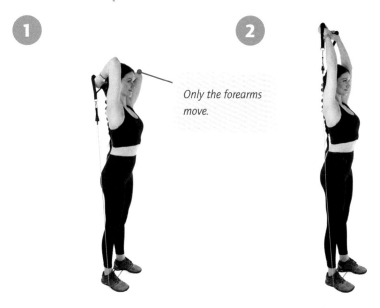

Only the forearms move.

- Stand upright and hold the band close to your head with both hands.

- As you exhale, extend your arms above your head.

- As you inhale, slowly lower your arms again. Make sure that your upper arms and elbows do not move. Only your forearms move.

- You can also perform the exercise while sitting.

Here you can see the video demo.

Triceps Kickback

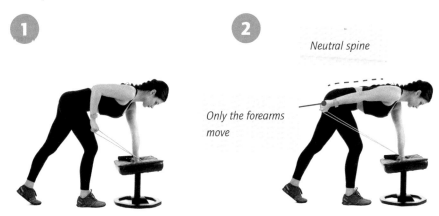

- Support yourself with one hand on an elevation (e.g., on a chair). This hand should be directly below the shoulder, and the band should be secured under the hand. Your other hand holds the band while the upper arm is parallel to the body, and the forearm points toward the floor. Make sure that your spine stays in its natural curve.

- As you exhale, stretch your free arm. Only the forearm moves. The upper arm and elbow do not move.

- As you inhale, bend your arm again. Repeat with your other arm.

Here you can see the video demo.

Narrow Push-Up

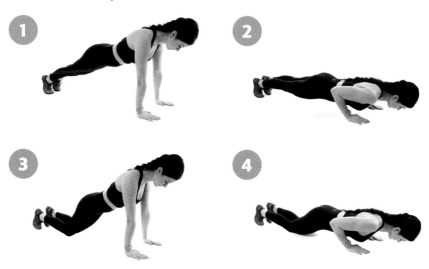

- In the prone position, straighten your body. Place your hands on the floor below your chest, slightly less than shoulder-width apart. Your fingers point forward, and your upper arms are very close to your body.

- As you exhale, straighten your arms, pushing your body up. The movement is initiated from your triceps and chest muscles.

- The weight is evenly distributed between your toes and hands. The head, neck, spine, glutes, and knees form a straight line, and the core is tight.

- As you inhale, bend your elbows again, and bring your body back down until you are just inches from the floor.

- If the exercise is too difficult for you, you can do it on your knees instead of your toes (see positions 3 and 4). Alternatively, you can place your upper body higher, for example, on the couch or even against the wall.

Here you can see the video demo.

WARM-UP

Arm Circles

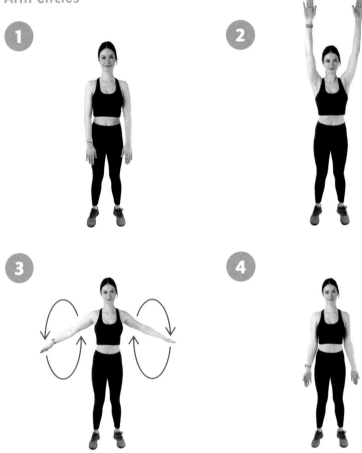

- Stand upright and lift your arms forward as you inhale.
- In a slow and controlled movement, make circles backward with both arms and lower your arms again as you exhale.

Here you can see the video demo.

Glute Bridge

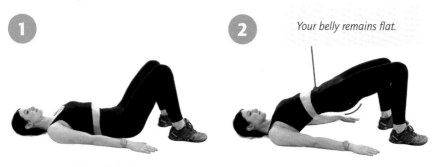

Your belly remains flat.

Squeeze your glutes hard.

- Lie on your back.

- As you exhale, push your hips up, squeezing your glutes as hard as possible in the highest position. Make sure your belly stays flat and does not bulge outward. Your knees should be directly above your ankles.

- As you inhale, lower your hips back down.

Here you can see the video demo.

Cuban Press With Very Light Weights

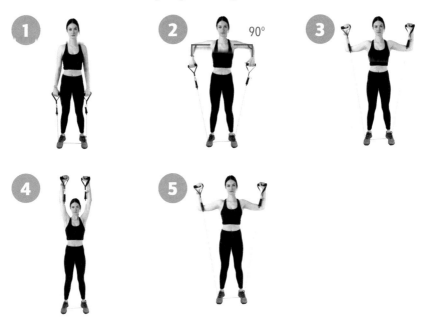

- Stand upright and hold a very light weight (or none at all) in your hands. The palms of your hands point backward.

- As you exhale, raise your upper arms to your sides until your elbows are bent at a 90-degree angle. The forearms hang down.

- As you inhale, rotate your arms so that your hands face up and your upper arms stay parallel to the floor.

- Press the weights over your head as you exhale.

- Finally, reverse the movement and return to the starting position.

- This is one repetition.

- For the warm-up, however, you don't have to lower your arms all the way down each time. It is enough to turn your forearms back down.

Here you can see the video demo.

Child's Pose Rocking

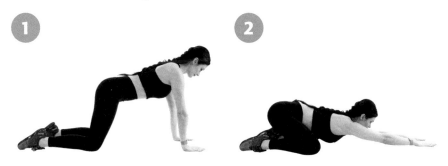

- Take a quadruped stance. As you exhale, bring your hips back until they land on your feet. As you do so, pull your arms forward and gently press your chest into the floor.

- As you inhale, come back to the quadruped position.

- Repeat the movement rocking back and forth.

Here you can see the video demo.

Hip and Knee Mobilization

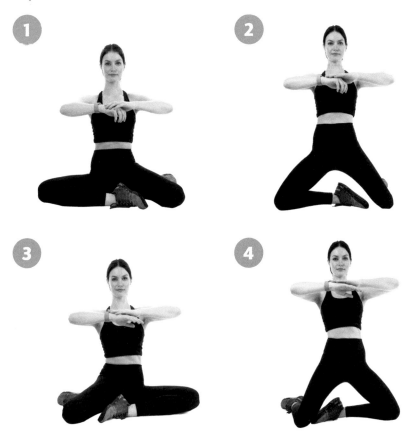

- Sit upright on the floor with your legs bent, and keep your back straight. For balance, you can bring your arms forward.

- As you exhale, come up onto your knees.

- As you inhale, slowly sit back down.

- Switch sides.

Here you can see the video demo.

Deep Squat With Ankle Rocking

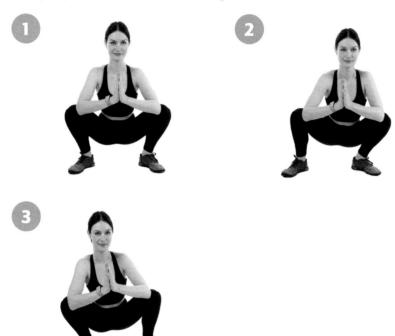

- Stand upright with your legs shoulder-width apart.

- As you inhale, slowly bend your knees and lower your hips. Lower your hips as far as possible while keeping your spine in its natural curve. Also, make sure that your knees do not collapse inward.

- Now, bring your hands together and push your knees further apart with your elbows.

- Hold this position, slowly rocking from side to side without lifting your feet off the floor.

Here you can see the video demo.

Wide Knee Child Pose (Lat and Chest Stretch and Hip Opener)

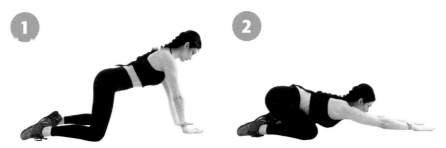

- Take a quadruped stance with your knees slightly wider apart. As you exhale, bring your hips back until they land on your feet. Pull your arms forward and gently press your chest into the floor as you do so.

- As you inhale, return to the quadruped position, and then bring your hips forward as far as possible to the floor.

- Repeat the movement rocking back and forth.

Here you can see the video demo.

Standing Chest Opener

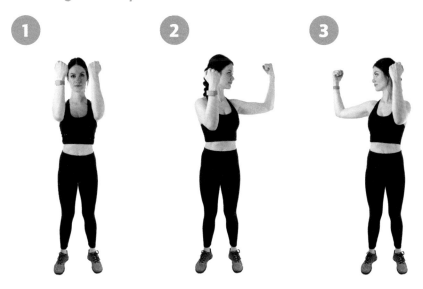

- Stand upright, arms raised and bent at 90 degrees.

- As you inhale, bring one bent arm to the side, following the movement of the arm with your head.

- As you exhale, bring your arm forward again. Repeat, alternating sides.

Here you can see the video demo.

Thread the Needle

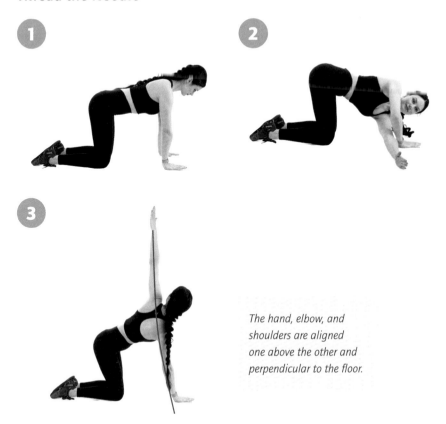

The hand, elbow, and shoulders are aligned one above the other and perpendicular to the floor.

- Take the quadruped stance.

- As you inhale, bring your arm up and open your chest. Your other hand, elbow, and shoulder should be aligned one above the other and perpendicular to the floor.

- As you exhale, bring your arm under your upper body, and rest your shoulder on the floor.

- Repeat with the other side.

Here you can see the video demo.

Banded Shoulder Circles

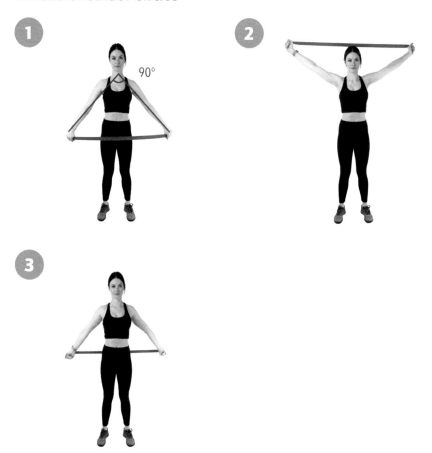

- Stand upright and take a long band in your hands so that your arms form a 90-degree angle and hang down at this angle.

- As you inhale, slowly bring the band back over your head as far as possible.

- As you exhale, bring the band back down to the front.

Here you can see the video demo.

Straight-Arm Shoulder Rotation

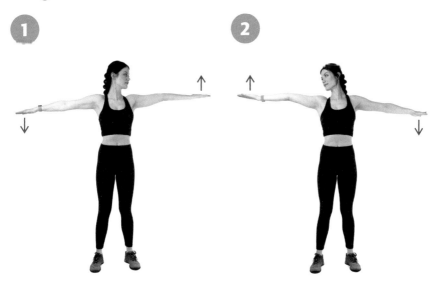

- Stand upright. Both arms are stretched out to the sides and parallel to the floor.

- Now turn your head in the direction of one arm. Turn the palm of the hand you look at upward and the palm of the other hand downward.

- Turn your head to the other hand while turning your palms the other way around.

Here you can see the video demo.

Standing Side Bend

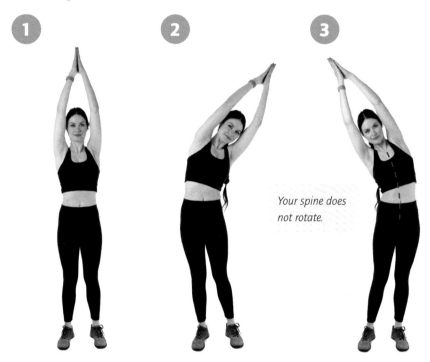

*Your spine does
not rotate.*

- Stand upright and bring your hands together above your head.

- As you exhale, slowly bend to one side. Make sure that your spine does not rotate.

- As you inhale, slowly straighten up again.

- Repeat with the other side.

Here you can see the video demo.

Body Weight Deep Squat

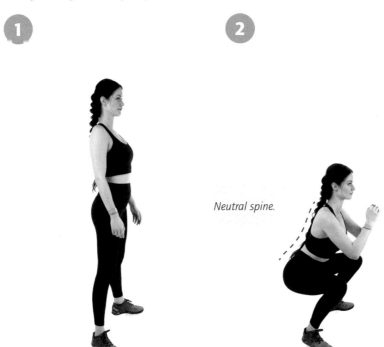

Neutral spine.

- Stand upright with your legs shoulder-width apart.

- As you inhale, slowly bend your knees and lower your hips. Lower your hips as far as possible while keeping your spine in its natural curve. Make sure that your knees do not collapse inward.

- As you exhale, push your body back up over the center of your foot.

Here you can see the video demo.

COOL-DOWN

Downward Facing Dog (Adho Mukha Svansasana)

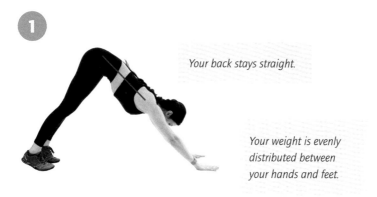

Your back stays straight.

Your weight is evenly distributed between your hands and feet.

- Stand hip-width apart. Your feet are pointing in the direction of your hands. Your weight is on your hands. Spread your fingers wide.

- As you exhale, push your hips up. At the same time, your back should remain straight, and your heel should be pressed into the floor as much as possible. Your neck is relaxed, and your weight is evenly distributed between your hands and feet.

- As you inhale, step out of the position.

Here you can see the video demo.

Upward Facing Dog (Urdhva Mukha Svanasana)

1

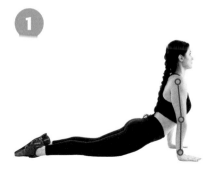

Your hands are under the shoulders and push your upper body up.

- As you inhale, straighten your arms, lifting your torso backward. The hands are just below the shoulders and push the upper body upwards.

- On the exhale, step out of the position.

Here you can see the video demo.

Biceps and Forearm Stretch

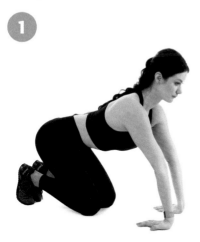

- Take the quadruped stance, placing your hands on the floor so your fingers point toward your legs. Breathe deeply.

Here you can see the video demo.

High Lunge

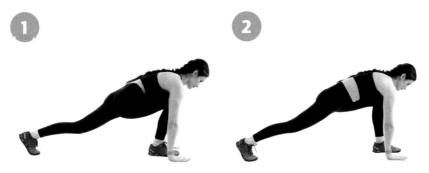

- **(From the Forward Bend)** As you inhale, stretch one leg far back and bend the front leg at the same time. Place your hands either side of the front foot.

- **(From the Downward Facing Dog)** As you inhale, bring your back foot forward between your hands.

- Your front leg is bent at 90 degrees, and your knee is placed right above your foot. Let your pelvis drop down.

Here you can see the video demo.

Seated Forward Bend

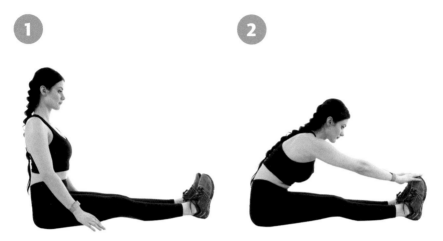

- Your legs are fully extended, and your upper body is upright.

- As you exhale, bend forward with your lower back as straight as possible. As you do so, push your tailbone back and try to bring your upper body as close to your thighs as possible.

- Breathe deeply during the stretch. On the exhale, step out of the position.

Here you can see the video demo.

Child Pose (Lat and Chest Stretch)

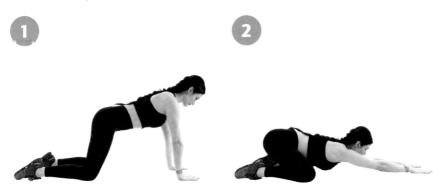

- Take the quadruped stance. As you exhale, bring your hips back until they land on your feet. Pull your arms forward and gently press your chest into the floor as you do so. Breathe deeply as you stretch.

Here you can see the video demo.

Supine Spinal Twist

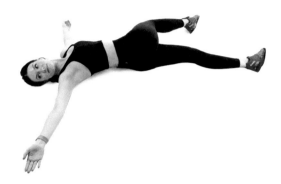

- Lie with your back flat on the floor. Your arms are stretched and lie relaxed on the floor either side of your body.

- Bend one leg and bring it to the side while exhaling. Meanwhile, turn your upper body and head to the other side. Breathe deeply while you are holding this position. Try to push the bent knee and opposite arm farther apart as you exhale, gently pressing them to the floor.

- As you inhale, straighten up again. Repeat on the other side.

Here you can see the video demo.

Side Deltoid Stretch

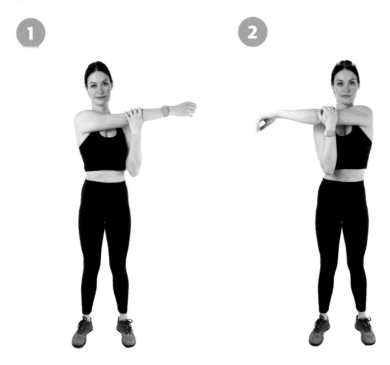

- Stretch one arm in front of your chest and hold it with the other arm. Gently stretch the shoulder of the gripped arm. Repeat on the other side.

Here you can see the video demo.

Mountain to Upward Salute Pose
(Tadasana to Urdhva Hastasana)

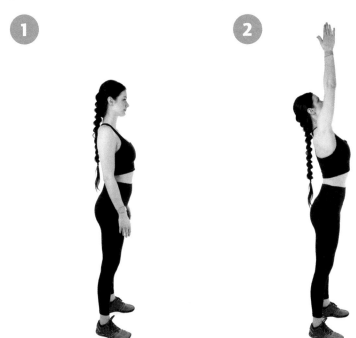

- "Tadasana" means mountain pose, and you simply stand straight and firm on the floor with a straightened and tall spine.

- As you inhale, bring your hands together above your head. Your eyes follow your hands, and the upper back bends slightly backward ("Urdhva Hastasana" = hands upward).

Here you can see the video demo.

Pigeon to Half Pigeon Pose to Single-Leg Forward Bend Pose

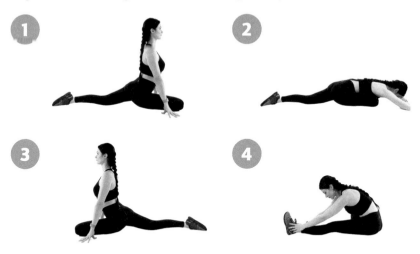

- Your front leg is bent at the knee, and the back leg is completely extended. Both legs should be in line. Straighten your upper body and bring your front leg in at a right angle.

- As you exhale, bend forward with your back straight and push your tailbone back. Rest your forehead on the floor, relax, and stretch your arms with your palms facing up. Breathe deeply as you stretch.

- As you exhale, return to the starting position and straighten your torso. Then rotate at your hips with your upper body at 180 degrees so that the bent leg that was previously in front touches the inside of the extended leg near the pubic bone with the foot.

- As you exhale, turn slightly toward the extended leg, and bend forward with your lower back as straight as possible. As you do this, push the tailbone back and try to bring your upper body as close to your thighs as possible.

- Breathe deeply during the stretch. Exhale as you come out of the position.

Here you can see the video demo.

Triceps Stretch

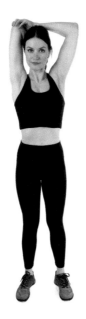 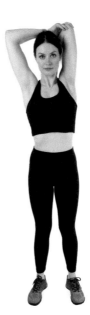

- Stand upright with legs shoulder-width apart. Bend your right arm with your elbow pointing to the ceiling and hand resting on your neck. With your left hand, gently press down on your right elbow until you feel a stretch.

- Breathe deeply as you stretch. Switch arms.

Here you can see the video demo.

Standing Forward Bend (Uttanasana)

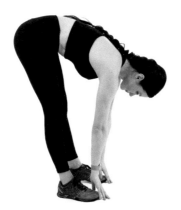

- As you exhale, bend your upper body forward. Pull your hamstrings and sit bones (ischium or pelvis) upward as you do so.

- Try to draw your shoulder blades toward your hips and place your hands flat on the floor. If necessary, you can bend your legs while doing this.

Here you can see the video demo.

Standing Forward Bend With Shoulder Opener

1

2

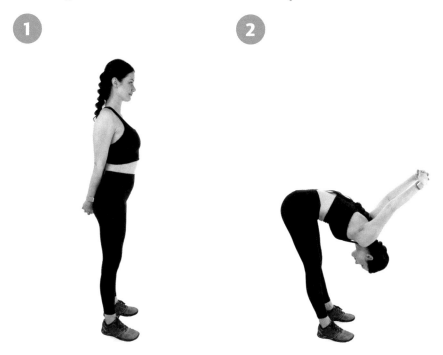

- Stand upright with your legs shoulder-width apart and clasp your hands behind your back.

- As you exhale, bend forward. As you do so, continue to bring your clasped hands forward over your head with your arms extended until they are parallel to the floor or as far as you can go. Breathe deeply as you stretch.

- As you inhale, straighten up again, and only then open your hands.

Here you can see the video demo.

REFERENCES

Apostolopoulos, N. C., Lahart, I. M., Plyley, M. J., Taunton, J., Nevill, A. M., Koutedakis Y., Wyon, M. & Metsios, G. S. (2018). The effects of different passive static stretching intensities on recovery from unaccustomed eccentric exercise – a randomized controlled trial. *Applied Physiology, Nnutrition, and Metabolism = Physiologie appliquee, nutrition et metabolisme, 43* (8), 806-815. https://doi.org/10.1139/apnm-2017-0841
https://pubmed.ncbi.nlm.nih.gov/29529387/

Astrup, A., Toubro, S., Cannon, S., Hein, P., Breum, L. & Madsen, J. (1990). Caffeine: A double-blind, placebo-controlled study of its thermogenic, metabolic, and cardiovascular effects in healthy volunteers. *The American Journal of Clinical Nutrition, 51* (5), 759-767. https://doi.org/10.1093/ajcn/51.5.759
https://pubmed.ncbi.nlm.nih.gov/2333832/

Ayyad, C. & Andersen, T. (2000). Long-term efficacy of dietary treatment of obesity: A systematic review of studies published between 1931 and 1999. *Obesity Reviews: An Official Journal of the International Association for the Study of Obesity, 1* (2), 113-119. https://doi.org/10.1046/j.1467-789x.2000.00019.x
https://pubmed.ncbi.nlm.nih.gov/12119984/

Baker, P. & Norton, L. (2019). *Fat loss forever: How to lose fat and KEEP it off.* Independently Published.

Berardi, J., Andrews, R., St. Pierre, B., Scott-Dixon, K., Kollias, H. & DePutter, C. (2019). *Nutrition: The complete guide (Edition 2).* Carpinteria: International Sports Sciences Association.

Contreras, B. & Cordoza, G. (2019). *GLUTE LAB: The art and science of strength and physique training.* Victory Belt Publishing.

Gropper, S. A. S., Smith, J. L. & Groff, J. L. (2009). *Advanced nutrition and human metabolism.* 5th ed. Australia; Belmont, CA: Wadsworth Cengage Learning.

Hill, C., Weir, B. W., Fuentes, L. W., Garcia-Alvarez, A., Anouti, D. P. & Cheskin, L. J. (2018). Relationship between weekly patterns of caloric intake and reported weight

loss outcomes: Retrospective cohort study. *JMIR mHealth and uHealth, 6* (4), e83. https://doi.org/10.2196/mhealth.8320
https://pubmed.ncbi.nlm.nih.gov/29661750/

Hsouna, H., Boukhris, O., Abdessalem, R., Trabelsi, K., Ammar, A., Shephard, R. J. & Chtourou, H. (2019). Effect of different nap opportunity durations on short-term maximal performance, attention, feelings, muscle soreness, fatigue, stress and sleep. *Physiology & Behavior, 211,* 112673. https://doi.org/10.1016/j.physbeh.2019.112673
https://pubmed.ncbi.nlm.nih.gov/31491444/

Jåbekk, P., Jensen, R. M., Sandell, M. B., Haugen, E., Katralen, L. M. & Bjorvatn, B. (2020). A randomized controlled pilot trial of sleep health education on body composition changes following 10 weeks' resistance exercise. *The Journal of Sports Medicine and Physical Fitness, 60* (5), 743-748. https://doi.org/10.23736/S0022-4707.20.10136-1
https://pubmed.ncbi.nlm.nih.gov/32141273/

Kellmann M. (2010). Preventing overtraining in athletes in high-intensity sports and stress/recovery monitoring. *Scandinavian Journal of Medicine & Science in Sports, 20 Suppl 2,* 95-102. https://doi.org/10.1111/j.1600-0838.2010.01192.x
https://pubmed.ncbi.nlm.nih.gov/20840567/

Kellmann, M., Bertollo, M., Bosquet, L., Brink, M., Coutts, A. J., Duffield, R., Erlacher, D., Halson, S. L., Hecksteden, A., Heidari, J., Kallus, K. W., Meeusen, R., Mujika, I., Robazza, C., Skorski, S., Venter, R. & Beckmann, J. (2018). Recovery and performance in sport: Consensus statement. *International Journal of Sports Physiology and Performance, 13* (2), 240-245. https://doi.org/10.1123/ijspp.2017-0759
https://pubmed.ncbi.nlm.nih.gov/29345524/

Kirschen, G. W., Jones, J. J. & Hale, L. (2020). The impact of sleep duration on performance among competitive athletes: A systematic literature review. *Clinical Journal of Sport Medicine: Official Journal of the Canadian Academy of Sport Medicine, 30* (5), 503-512. https://doi.org/10.1097/JSM.0000000000000622
https://pubmed.ncbi.nlm.nih.gov/29944513/

Langeveld, M. & de Vries, J. H. (2013). Het magere resultaat van diëten [The mediocre results of dieting]. *Nederlands Tijdschrift voor Geneeskunde, 157* (29), A6017.
https://pubmed.ncbi.nlm.nih.gov/23859104/

Meule A. (2020). The Psychology of Food Cravings: the Role of Food Deprivation. *Current nutrition reports, 9* (3), 251–257. https://doi.org/10.1007/s13668-020-00326-0
https://pubmed.ncbi.nlm.nih.gov/32578025/

Pérez-Gómez, J., Adsuar, J. C., Alcaraz, P. E. & Carlos-Vivas, J. (2020). Physical exercises for preventing injuries among adult male football players: A systematic review. *Journal of Sport and Health Science,* S2095-2546(20)30152-6. Advance online publication. https://doi.org/10.1016/j.jshs.2020.11.003
https://pubmed.ncbi.nlm.nih.gov/33188962/

Precision Nutrition Inc. *Never press "pause" on your health and fitness again. This free tool is your secret weapon. Use this genius dial to keep making progress – no matter how tough your day ... or week ... or month.* Unter: https://www.precisionnutrition.com/pause-button-mentality-infographic
Schöps, I. (2008). Yoga: *Das große Praxisbuch für Einsteiger & Fortgeschrittene.* Bath: Parragon Books Ltd.

U.S. Department of Agriculture, Agricultural Research Service (2019). *FoodData Central.* fdc.nal.usda.gov.

Vivanti A. P. (2012). Origins for the estimations of water requirements in adults. *European Journal of Clinical Nutrition, 66* (12), 1282-1289. https://doi.org/10.1038/ejcn.2012.157
https://pubmed.ncbi.nlm.nih.gov/23093341/

Watson A. M. (2017). Sleep and athletic performance. *Current Sports Medicine Reports, 16* (6), 413-418. https://doi.org/10.1249/JSR.0000000000000418
https://pubmed.ncbi.nlm.nih.gov/29135639/

All links were checked on 02/14/2021.

Credits

Cover photo: James Patrick Photography; courtesy of Elena Biedert

Cover design: Anja Elsen

Layout: Anja Elsen

Interior photos: Tobias Serf, Tobias Serf Photography; courtesy of Elena Biedert

Managing editor: Elizabeth Evans

Copy editor: Sarah Tomblin, www.sarahtomblinediting.com

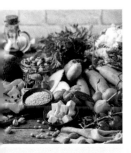

BEST IN NUTRITION

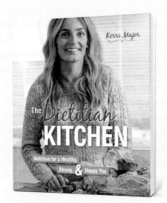

ISBN 978-1-78255-184-3
$22.95 US

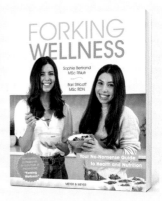

ISBN 978-1-78255-209-3
$24.95 US

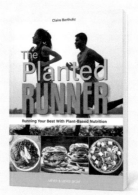

ISBN 978-1-78255-246-8
$24.95 US

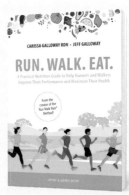

ISBN 978-1-78255-261-1
$19.95 US

MEYER & MEYER Sport
Von-Coels-Str. 390
52080 Aachen
Germany

Phone   +49 02 41 - 9 58 10 - 13
Fax   +49 02 41 - 9 58 10 - 10
E-Mail   sales@m-m-sports.com
Website www.m-m-sports.com

MEYER
& MEYER
SPORT

BEST IN FITNESS

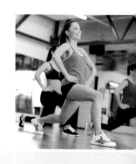

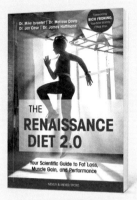

ISBN 978-1-78255-190-4
$26.95 US

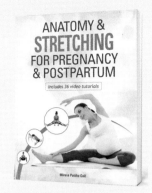

ISBN 978-1-78255-255-0
$26.95 US

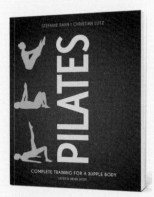

ISBN 978-1-78255-186-7
$29.95 US

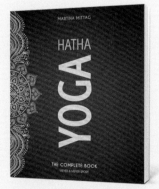

ISBN 978-1-78255-185-0
$34.95 US

MEYER & MEYER Sport
Von-Coels-Str. 390
52080 Aachen
Germany

Phone
Fax
E-Mail
Website

+49 02 41 - 9 58 10 - 13
+49 02 41 - 9 58 10 - 10
sales@m-m-sports.com
www.m-m-sports.com

MEYER
& MEYER
SPORT